Knife, Fire
and
Boiling Oil

WILLIAM JOHN BISHOP was highly regarded as a librarian, editor
and historian both in Britain and abroad. After more than thirty
years in libraries he decided to devote the remainder of his life
to his own researches in medical bibliography and history. He
was editor of *Medical History*, the only British journal devoted
to the history of medicine. In 1959 he was elected an honorary
member of the Royal Society of Medicine. He died in 1961.

Knife, Fire
and
Boiling Oil

The Early History of Surgery

W.J. BISHOP

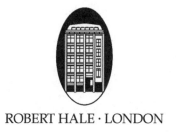

ROBERT HALE · LONDON

© W.J. Bishop 1960
First published in Great Britain 1960
This paperback edition published 2010

ISBN 978-0-7090-9155-4

Robert Hale Limited
Clerkenwell House
Clerkenwell Green
London EC1R 0HT

www.halebooks.com

The right of W.J. Bishop to be identified as author
of this work has been asserted by him in accordance
with the Copyright, Designs and Patents Act 1988

A catalogue record for this book is available from the British Library

2 4 6 8 10 9 7 5 3 1

Printed in the UK by the MPG Books Group, Bodmin and King's Lynn

CONTENTS

ILLUSTRATIONS

ACKNOWLEDGMENT

Grateful acknowledgment is made to Dr. E. Ashworth Underwood, Director of the Wellcome Historical Medical Museum, who supplied the illustrations for this book.

PREFACE

THE brilliant achievements of modern surgery have been brought home to every man, not only by the numerous excellent books which have been written on the subject but also by the Press, the cinema, radio and television. The two events which mark the beginning of "modern" surgery are the introduction of anaesthesia and of the antiseptic system. Surgical anaesthesia did not come into general use until some years after the clear demonstration of the anaesthetic properties of ether in 1846 and the antiseptic system was still struggling for acceptance in the eighteen-seventies and 'eighties. Modern surgery is therefore not much more than a century old.

While it is, broadly speaking, true that the most junior house surgeon of today is better equipped to treat a surgical condition than any of the great master surgeons of the past, it is often forgotten that medical history is—like that of all arts and sciences—continuous. Present-day knowledge and techniques have not come into being suddenly, but have resulted from the cumulative observations and experiments of centuries. In the year 1362 Guy de Chauliac, the leading surgeon of the fourteenth century, completed a great textbook of surgery. In the prologue to this work he acknowledged the debt which he owed to his predecessors and said: "We are like children standing on the shoulders of a giant, for we can see all that the giant can see, and a little more."

It is the purpose of this book to tell something of the giants who paved the way for the triumphs of modern surgery and of the conditions under which they worked.

CHAPTER ONE

The Dawn of Surgery

THE history of disease is much older than that of mankind. Fossilized bacteria similar to those responsible for many infections that afflict man today have been found in geological formations that are 500 million years old. Fossil shells dating from an era almost equally remote show unmistakable evidence of disturbance by injury and by parasites. Examination of the skeletons of dinosaurs and other great reptiles that roamed the earth millions of years ago show that these creatures suffered from fractures, bone tumours, arthritis, osteomyelitis, dental caries and other diseases that still constitute medical problems. The available evidence is limited to the changes that can be observed in bone and teeth, but it is safe to assume that disease processes were equally prevalent in the soft organs and tissues of these prehistoric monsters. The general pattern of disease has not changed in essentials during the millions of years that life has existed on this planet.

Man has been subject to disease from the time of his first appearance on the stage of prehistory some 500,000 years ago. The human body has been constantly exposed to assault and injury, to invasion by parasites, to extremes of heat and cold, and to infections. It is probable that early man suffered from a number of diseases due to nutritional factors and to disorders of the body chemistry, but we have no direct evidence of this. In the case of cancer, we are on surer ground. Pithecanthropus, the Java ape-man discovered in 1891 and considered to be half a million years old, had a morbid growth on his femur, and it is probable that bone and other forms of cancer have existed from the earliest times. The remains of Neanderthal man, who roamed through Europe, Africa and the Near East in the last glacial period, showed clear evidence of arthritis and of suppurative bone disease. When we come to the New Stone Age the evidence of the bones is even more revealing: we find that

Neolithic man suffered from arthritis, sinusitis, tumours, congenital dislocations and fractures, and tuberculosis of the spine.

The only conclusion that can be drawn from this evidence is that disease has always been an inseparable companion of life. In considering the question of what our earliest ancestors did about disease we are on very uncertain ground. At the remotest periods the evidence which we have only proves that disease existed; it tells us nothing about the way in which early man reacted to his afflictions. Certain conclusions can, however, be drawn from evidence in the late prehistoric period and from a study of the medicine and magic of primitive peoples.

A distinction has to be drawn between internal diseases and those external diseases which are commonly regarded as being surgical in their nature. With regard to internal disease there is abundant evidence indicating that early man did not admit the existence of disease from what we call natural causes. He regarded such disease as being the result of the malevolent influence exercised by a supernatural being or by a human enemy. Among primitive peoples it is a common belief that disease is caused by the loss of something essential to life. The "spirit" or "soul" leaves the body at death and during sleep; what more natural than to think that it can be enticed away from the body by black magic. Disease is also thought to be caused by projection of some morbid material or influence into the victim. In treating disease due to the loss of the soul, the medicine-man falls into a trance and sends his own soul to find that of the patient. When he emerges from his trance he exhibits some object, such as a pebble or a bead, containing the soul, and this is rubbed on the head of the patient. The projection of disease from a distance is well known among the Aborigines of Central Australia and is manifested in the ritual called the "Pointing of the Bone". A long slender stick is pointed towards the victim to the accompaniment of a chant or spell. The bone or stick is then buried in secret. As soon as the victim learns that he has been "boned" he invariably falls ill and he may die of sheer fright. A case of this kind which occurred in Australia a few years ago attracted world-wide publicity because the victim was eventually saved after many months of hospitalization. That severe and often fatal illnesses can be induced by these methods is an undoubted fact, and it is equally incontestible that the primitive medicine-man often effects remarkable cures by means which are basically indistinguishable from those employed by the most up-to-date medical psychologist.

The situation with regard to injuries and external diseases is rather different. A wound, a bruise, a fracture, or a foreign body such as an arrow-head or a thorn are tangible things and they demand attention. The art of surgery originated under the compelling influence of some immediate crisis. Our earliest ancestors were isolated in a hostile world and were obliged to carry on a ceaseless struggle to obtain food and shelter and to protect themselves from their enemies. The first men quickly became familiar with the sight of wounds. One of the first things that a wounded man would do, whatever the nature of his injury, would be to protect it from the influence of external forces or agents. For this there was, and is to this day, only one means—the application of a dressing. From amongst the great variety of substances available in his immediate surroundings, the injured man was rapidly led to exercise a choice. The first dressing ever used may have been the leaf of a tree or shrub. Some substances were found to be less painful when applied than others; some gave better and more secure protection. Many observations were made, many things tried, and in time a body of experience was accumulated and was passed on orally to others for use in similar emergencies. The first results were modified by daily use and experiment and a considerable body of inherited knowledge gradually came into being. The art of dressing wounds long constituted the whole of medicine; the use of internal remedies, herbs, etc., and that of the knife or of fire came much later. Some light on the methods by which early man treated wounds is provided by a study of present-day primitive and folk medicine.

Haemorrhage, that most acute of all emergencies for the first-aider, calls for immediate action. Some primitive peoples developed quite effective methods to control bleeding. The use of cobwebs upon a bleeding wound is a very ancient folk remedy, and is referred to by Shakespeare in *A Midsummer Night's Dream*, where he makes Bottom say to Cobweb:

"I shall desire you of more acquaintance, good
    Master Cobweb:
If I cut my finger I shall make bold with you."

It has been stated that at the time of the battle of Crécy
(26 August, 1346) the English soldiers carried boxes containing
spiders' webs as first-aid equipment. This practice may have
had some basis in that the presence of a fine filament, such as
a spider's web, would facilitate coagulation of the blood; but it
would also seem to carry some danger from the point of view of
infection.

Among some Northern peoples snow is laid on a bleeding
wound. The North American Indians, on the other hand, often
applied hot leaves or packed the wound with hot sand, with
eagles' down or with scrapings from the inside of tanned hides.
In certain cases they cauterized wounds with a hot brand. As
they usually kept wounds clean and treated their wounded in
isolated lodges, they often obtained better results than the
white man. The Melanesians applied a bandage of tapa cloth
tightly to the bleeding part. The cautery or hot iron was used
to control haemorrhage in many parts of the world. The only
tribe known to ligate blood vessels (with tendons) is the Masai.

The natives of Victoria, Australia, looked upon bleeding
with favour as it cleansed the wound. They were in the habit
of encouraging the flow by suction, by changes in posture and
kneading the tissues. When the wound had been sufficiently
purified by these means they laid upon it a lump of resin as a
dressing. The same tribe are said to have been aware of the
danger of retained wound secretions and when the lips of a
wound closed prematurely they would open them up again.
The Dacota Indians seem to have used drainage, inserting
wicks of soft tree bark into their wounds. They also washed them
out with a kind of syringe made of a bladder and the quill of
a feather.

The suturing of wounds was practised by some primitive
peoples and may not have been unknown to prehistoric man.
Bone needles furnished with an eye, together with the tools used
in their manufacture, have been found in palaeolithic deposits
both in France and in England. They were made by taking a

splinter from a bone by means of a graver and then rounding it by scraping with a serrated flint. Some Indian tribes suture with threads of sinew or bone needles; the needles are left in and the thread twisted round them—a kind of skewer method which was, incidentally, still used in operations for the cure of harelip as late as the eighteenth century.

One of the most extraordinary methods of suturing wounds, especially abdominal wounds, is by means of termites or ants. This method has been observed in such widely separated places as India, East Africa and Brazil. It consists in bringing the edges of the wound close together and allowing the termites to bite through them. The powerful jaws of the insect act like pincers or like the metal clips (Michel clips) used in modern surgery and keep the edges of the wound in close apposition. The bodies of the insects are then cut off.

By way of dressings fresh leaves are sometimes applied and sometimes a kind of poultice made of herbs or the soft bark of trees is laid upon the wound. Clay was employed for this purpose by the Blacks of Australia and tar is an old and favourite folk dressing in Europe.

Two African tribes, the Masai and the Akamba, suture by means of thorns. Long white thorns of the acacia are passed through the skin and muscular tissue well back from the border of the wound and out through the opposite side. A path for the thorn is made by means of a sharp awl. A strip of tough vegetable fibre or bass is then wound around the protruding edges of the thorn in a figure of eight. The surfaces of the wound are thus brought fairly well together and the edges of the skin are then more carefully pierced with the awl and brought neatly together by a series of closely set separate stitches, each tied with a reef knot. Sword slashes and spear stabs sewn up in this way often do well, despite the absence of drainage.

The treatment of the terrible wounds inflicted by assegai, swords, and knobkerries was often heroic. After washing with the juice of certain leaves, a heated spear might be thrust into a wound to burn away unhealthy tisue and stop bleeding. A less painful but nevertheless crude method of wound treatment was by clapping on a poultice of cow dung and dust. Barbed arrows were pushed through and drawn out on the other side

of the body if possible; otherwise the protruding end of the
arrow was tied to a sprung sapling which was then released,
jerking out the missile.

David Livingstone, being a qualified surgeon, naturally took
a special interest in African medicine and he left descriptions of
many remarkable native practices. On one of his journeys he
saw a woman who had an arrow-head embedded in her back
just below the ribs, penetrating the left lung. Although several
inches of the barbed arrow were embedded in the flesh near
the diaphragm, and air was coming out of the wound, the
native surgeon did not hesitate to cut out the arrow with a
portion of the lung. The woman recovered. On another occasion
Livingstone witnessed an extraordinary method of treating a
gunshot wound with fracture of the bones of the leg. A hole
two feet deep and four feet long was dug in the ground and
the wounded man was sat in it with his legs outstretched. The
legs were covered by leaves, earth and mud, over which a fire
of sticks and grass was built. The fire was allowed to burn until
the heat had penetrated to the buried limb and could no longer
be borne. The patient was then taken out of the hole, and the
injured leg was stretched, splinted and tightly bound.

In skull fractures African natives remove any piece of loose
bone and bind certain leaves over the part. Bullets are occasionally removed, a stiff hair from an elephant's tail being
used as a probe and the missile being worked out through the
original opening by massage and pinching. A man gored in the
abdomen by an elephant replaced the bowels, which had been
partially torn out, inserted a small calabash to keep them in
place, then drew the skin over all and sewed it across. The
shape of the calabash could be clearly seen, but the man recovered and was able to undertake the hardest labour.

Among the Berbers and Shawiya of Algeria the following substances are applied to wounds, especially to control bleeding:
ashes of rag or of paper, pieces of dirty wool dipped in olive oil,
powdered green leaves or a species of nightshade, the fresh
leaves or bark of the walnut tree, dried goats' dung, damp earth
(which must be good since we are sprung from it) and powdered
gallnut. It may be noted that their preference for dirty wool is
one which they shared with many European surgeons even as

late as the nineteenth century. In the same way hands and instruments are washed *after* use in any water, hot or cold, clean or dirty, which is available. Red-hot cutting instruments are sometimes used, but solely with the idea of checking haemorrhage.

Bullet wounds are often left alone when deep, but some surgeons dress the wound by inserting into it, with the aid of a probe, a rag steeped in honey and alum. The rag is left in the wound and this dressing is renewed daily for five days, at the end of which time the wound should be ready to respond to a surface dressing. Butter or a mixture of butter and honey are commonly introduced into bullet wounds by means of a European syringe or by the old-time native instruments, which consist of a tube of oleander wood, narrow at one end but extending to a bell-mouth at the other. A commonly used surface dressing is a mixture of acetate of copper, sulphide of copper and ammonium chloride, powdered and boiled in honey to form a paste. Dusting powders for application to cuts are made from a variety of dried and powdered leaves, alone or mixed with alum, and also from the larvae of a certain beetle. Other ointments for suppurating wounds and sores are made up as follows:

Six parts of the dregs of red vinegar boiled over a charcoal fire with six parts of honey, and mixed with one part of copper acetate.

Olive oil boiled with a quarter of a cupful of fat from a goat's kidney, one-fifth of a cupful of yellow candle grease, one-sixth of a cupful of acetate of copper, and a piece of aloes as large as a thimble.

Honey heated till it simmers with equal parts of red vinegar, acetate of copper, myrrh and aloes.

Fractures and dislocations account for a very large proportion of all injuries and it is possible that Neolithic man was familiar with methods of splinting by means of sticks or pieces of bark. There is no evidence that this was actually done in the Neolithic period but the men of the New Stone Age were skilled craftsmen and, as they were able to carry out such formidable procedures as trepanation, it is reasonable to suppose they had hit upon the idea of stretching a broken limb and fixing it in position. Well-healed fractures have certainly been observed in the bones of prehistoric man, but these cannot all have resulted from surgical intervention. Fractures occur frequently among wild animals and a relatively large percentage of these fractures heal spontaneously with good functional results. We do know that some primitive peoples developed very clever methods of immobilizing a fractured limb. The Shoshone Indians made a splint of fresh raw hide that had been soaked in water. It could be adjusted very accurately and when it had dried it made an effective cast. In the case of a compound fracture a window was sometimes cut into the cast to allow drainage. Other tribes used splints of wood or bark and fixed them carefully with bandages. Splints were sometimes left on until the fracture united, but as the necessary extension was not provided, the results were not always satisfactory. Some South Australian tribes made splints of clay which, when they dried, were as good as plaster of Paris. Others simply applied slats of wood fastened by thongs. Bone-setting was practised as a specialty in many tribes. With regard to minor surgery there are among native races three methods of blood letting: direct venesection, scarification, with or without the use of "cupping" glasses, and the application of leeches. Venesection—the direct opening of a vein—is practised by many uncivilized races. Some South American Indians are said to do it by shooting a small arrow from a bow into different parts of the body until a vein is pierced—a method that probably has some magical significance. The Incas of Peru are said to have opened veins as close as possible to the site of the pain. In the case of severe headache they bled themselves between the eyebrows using a flint attached to a stick.

Scarification consists in making a number of superficial incisions to promote bleeding. Among native races the instruments used are knives, sharp mussel shells, flints, glass, thorns and fish bones. Scarification preceded by suction constituted what was known as "wet cupping". Cups were made of glass, metal or horn. A common method of performing the operation was to stick dried flax to the bottom of the cup. The flax was ignited and when it was burning well the cup was clapped on the patient and left for about half an hour. The rarefied air had the effect of drawing blood to the part, which was then scarified. Sometimes scarification was carried out first and this was followed by suction, as among the Dacota and Canadian Indians. The Baganda of Central Africa, who have a great belief in blood-letting, practise this simple method: the site of operation—it is commonly the back of the head or neck or the shoulder—is first of all scarified with a razor. A small antelope or goat horn that has a hole pierced at the tip is then taken and its mouth is placed over the incisions. The blood-letter sucks hard through the tip of the horn. The blood of the patient is prevented from entering the mouth of the man who operates by a wad or coil of banana leaf fitted inside the horn. In "dry cupping" suction was used without scarification of the skin. Wounds and insect and snake bites were treated in this way with the object of drawing out the poisonous matter.

Leeches have been used for drawing blood from time immemorial. They were applied to every part of the body, but were especially convenient for extracting blood from places where the knife could not well be used and in the case of young children. Normally they would be left until fully gorged, when they would fall off. If it was necessary to remove them before they had done, salt was sprinkled on them; if required to suck after becoming fully gorged, their tails were cut off.

Cauterization—the use of hot irons or brands—has been practised from early times and for a great variety of conditions. The Bhils, a primitive race of Rajputana, employ the actual cautery for all diseases attended by swelling. The operators are said to be women. This barbarous method was, however, most commonly used to arrest haemorrhage or to remove dead flesh.

The great authority on African life, the late Sir Harry Johnston, recorded many examples of surgical skill. He states that the Bantu surgeons, in cases of inflammation of the lungs or pleurisy, punch a hole in the chest until the air escapes through it. They dress the wound with butter and seem to have good results. Sir Harry also vouches for the fact that in abdominal wounds, extruded viscera were held in place by a gourd or shell over which the skin was sewn. Such cases often did well.

Apart from the treatment of wounds and injuries, there are records of operations being performed for a number of miscellaneous conditions. There is no doubt that enlarged neck glands were removed by some African native doctors in cases of sleeping sickness (trypanosomiasis). Neck tumours are cauterized in Rhodesia; the Galla and the Akamba remove the uvula; the Masai scarify inflamed tonsils and operate on abscesses of the liver and spleen; temporary collapse of the lung (artificial pneumothorax) and drainage of pus from the chest are practised in Uganda.

The native races of the Pacific were acquainted with most of the surgical methods which have been mentioned, and they possessed some techniques of their own. According to the Rev. William Ellis, author of *Polynesian Researches* (1833), some of their surgery was marked by "a rude promptness, temerity, and barbarism almost incredible". A man one day fell from a tree and dislocated some part of his neck. "His companions, on perceiving it, instantly took him up: one of them placed his head between his own knees, and held it firmly; while the others, taking hold of his body, twisted the joint into its proper place." A method not recommended in any Red Cross or St. John manual! On another occasion a young man who was carrying a large stone injured his back. He was laid flat on his face on the grass: one fellow grasped and pulled his shoulders, another his legs, while a third knelt upon his back and pressed his whole weight upon the spot where the spine appeared to be displaced. This unorthodox method of treating a slipped disk appears to have been successful because the injured man was soon able to resume his work.

There is evidence for the performance of one major operation by men of the New Stone Age. This is the daring operation of trephination. This remarkable operation consisting in making perforations in the skull and removing disks of bone. When the first trephined skulls were found in France as early as 1685 it was assumed that the holes in them had been caused by wounds, but as many more skulls were excavated in various parts of the world, including Britain, doubts began to be expressed on this theory. For many years it seemed incredible that such a dangerous operation could have been carried out without any form of anaesthesia and with the flint and bone tools that were the Neolithic surgeons' only instruments. Experiments performed on skulls after death showed, however, that it was not only possible but relatively easy to trephine a skull with a large flint. It has now been established that there were three different techniques: by patiently scratching the bone, by making a circular incision that was gradually deepened, or by drilling a series of small holes arranged in a circle and then cutting the bridges between them. The formation of new tissue at the cut edges shows that many individuals survived the operation and, incredible as it may seem, some skulls were trephined as many as five or six times. Hundreds of trephined skulls have now been examined. Examples dating from the Neolithic period have been found in the Western Mediterranean area, in Spain, Portugal, Algiers and Italy, in Great Britain, Switzerland, Germany, Austria, France, Belgium, Denmark, Sweden, Poland and Russia. Primitive trephining was also practised in North and South America but principally in Peru and Mexico. The operation is still performed by native healers in parts of the Balkans, among some North African tribes, and in a number of primitive tribes of the Pacific.

The operation was usually practised on the parietal bone, sometimes on the frontal and occipital bones. The operator apparently knew that cutting through the sagittal suture would inevitably lead to fatal haemorrhage. Some perforations are small, others very large, and multiple perforations have been found, particularly in American material.

The reason for the performance of this operation has been the subject of endless debate. Some authorities believe it was originally carried out to make an opening in the head so that the evil spirit or diseased demon could escape. Support is lent to this theory by the fact that few trephined skulls show any signs of fracture or other injury and that the roundels of bone removed at operation were preserved and worn as charms or talismans. The second explanation is that the operation was entirely rational and that it was performed in cases of cranial injury to remove blood and splinters and so relieve compression. The question is complicated by the fact that a number of primitive peoples perform the operation of trephination to this day, but they apparently practise it for both reasons. Sometimes it is done for ritual purposes, but at other times for headache, vertigo, epilepsy and similar disorders, as well as for head injuries. But whatever the motives that led prehistoric man to perform this operation, perform it he did; and it is one of the most extraordinary things in the whole history of medicine that this operation which one usually associates with the modern brain surgeon should have been carried out by our pre-historic ancestors.

We have a very full description of the technique of trephining as carried out by the natives of Blanche Bay, New Britain. In the case of this people the operation was definitely carried out for the treatment of fractures of the skull, a very common injury resulting from the use of the sling-stones employed in inter-tribal warfare. The operation was usually performed on the frontal or parietal regions but sometimes on the occipital. The selection of cases for treatment was made by "the one who is skilled in healing". Those who had sustained extensive damage to the brain were not treated. The surgeon's instruments consisted of a knife made from a piece of bamboo, shaped to provide a double cutting edge; a scraper, an irregularly shaped piece of igneous rock with sharp edges; a blow-pipe, a hollow cylinder of bamboo; forceps made by doubling over a narrow strip of bamboo; a scoop made from a piece of coconut shell; needles made from sharpened hollow wing-bones of the flying-fox; and thread, double-plied threads made from banana fibre.

The operator carefully washed the wound with coconut milk and then made a triangular incision over the site of the fracture. He scraped away the tissues with the stone scraper, coconut milk being continuously poured over the wound. Then he blew inside the wound with a blow pipe, in an attempt to locate the spicules of bone; it was thought that the semi-conscious patient felt more pain when the current of air impinged on the fragments. These were picked out with the forceps while scraping and blowing were continued until all pieces were removed. An elaborate dressing composed of banana leaves, pepper, lime and young betelnut was placed in position. If the operator found that the brain was slightly damaged, he had no hesitation in scooping out the injured portion. After operation the patient was not disturbed for three days except to be given some soft food. The dressings were then removed and if pus was found the sutures were removed, the operation repeated and fresh dressings applied. A graphic description of trephination in New Britain was given by the Rev. J. A. Crump, a missionary who had spent many years in the South Seas. The man who performed the operation was the medicine-man or wizard of the tribe. He used a piece of shell or a flake of obsidian for a trephine. An incision was made over the seat of the fracture, generally in the shape of a Y or V and then perhaps some loose fragments were picked out with the fingernail, and while the assistants held back the scalp the fractured bone was scraped, cut and picked away, leaving the brain exposed to the size of a half-crown. All loose pieces having been removed, the scalp was carefully laid down and the wound bandaged. The patient was generally insensible from the time of the injury. In five or six days the bandages were removed and complete recovery resulted in two or three weeks. The number of deaths was said to be about twenty per cent and most of these resulted from the initial injury and not from any complication of the operation.

A similar description has been given by R. Parkinson, a German surveyor, of operations which he witnessed in New Britain. Among this people the instruments used were a splinter of obsidian, a sharp shark's tooth, or a mussel shell. The operator washed his hands and irrigated the wound with coconut milk. A diagonal incision was made across the site of the injury and a thin rattan rope was made fast to a lock of hair. The scalp covering was then slowly and carefully drawn back. Any loose splinters were carefully drawn out until the brain was visible. The operator then scraped around the opening in the roof of the skull so that all sharp corners were removed and the hole was round or elliptical. The opening in the skull was then covered with a piece of mal (a kind of paste made by beating a small branch of a tree from which the bark had been stripped) or with a small piece of the heart leaf of a certain banana which had been held over a glowing fire. The flesh was then carefully pulled over the skull and a net made of strips of rattan was drawn over it. An old native gave Parkinson an account of thirty-one cases, twenty-three of which had survived. Many of the patients were presented to Parkinson and one of them had been trephined twice.

Dr. E. Ford, who has reviewed the subject of trephination in Melanesia, states that "the circular opening might easily be taken for the handiwork of a modern European surgeon". The technique is not rigidly uniform in different parts of the Pacific, but it differs slightly with the district, the type of case, and the operator. What is extremely interesting is that the operation is only attempted for definite surgical purposes. According to Parkinson some operators in New Ireland have advanced beyond trephination for cases of fracture and use it for other illnesses and to relieve pain. What is very striking about all the descriptions of trephination as performed by primitive peoples is the high degree of surgical judgment shown in the selection of cases for operative intervention and the fact that the steps of the operation are carried out in an orderly manner. Great ingenuity is shown in devising instruments from the simplest materials, and there is rational nursing. Equally striking are the results, which, according to many accounts, surpassed those of many European operators in the nineteenth century. A series of thirty-two trephinations carried out at St. George's and Guy's Hospitals during the period 1870–77 carried a mortality of seventy-five per cent; the primitive native surgeons of Melanesia could claim over seventy per cent of survivals. There is little evidence as to the frequency of mental disturbance or epilepsy following such operations by primitive peoples, but it does not seem likely that such complications were more frequent than they are in the case of head injuries observed in our modern hospitals.

It is interesting to note that this very advanced surgery still retains some elements of magic. The primitive trephiner is usually the wizard or healer of the tribe, the man of power invested with all the prestige of the priest-physician. Charms were sometimes hung on the patient in order to promote healing, and the pieces of bone removed from the skull were carefully preserved as objects of magical significance.

Apart from trephination, Neolithic surgeons carried out

another cranial operation, the so-called Sincipital T. This procedure, which seems to have been carried out only on female skulls, consisted of a T-shaped scar beginning on the frontal bone, running along the sagittal suture and branching into two parts along the posterior edge of the parietal bones. A few skulls have been found with straight lines or oval cicatrices. The scars may have been caused by deep incision through the scalp or possibly by cauterization. It is not known whether the operation was performed for therapeutic, or for magico-religious ends, or possibly as a punishment. Oval scars have been found on skulls of the Guanches, early inhabitants of the Canary Islands, who made large scarifications with their stone knives on the part affected and then cauterized the wound with roots of malacca cane dipped in boiling grease (preference being given to the use of goats' grease). According to the Greek historian Herodotus (fifth century B.C.), it was the practice of many Libyan nomads "to take their children when four years old and with grease of sheeps' wool to burn the veins of their scalps and sometimes of their temples, that so the children may be never afterwards afflicted by phlegm running down from the head. They say this makes their children most healthy." The Greek surgeons of Alexandria made deep scarifications of the forehead in the treatment of eye diseases, and cauterization of the scalp was practised by Arabic physicians in the treatment of epilepsy and other nervous diseases. It is interesting to find that deep cauterizations of the head similar to those described by Herodotus were employed by the natives of the Loyalty Islands in the South Seas as late as 1874.

There are among the many prehistoric cave paintings existing in Europe a number of representations of human hands from which one or more fingers or parts of fingers are missing. These pictures have led some writers to assert that amputation of the fingers was practised in prehistoric times, probably as part of some sacrificial or propitiatory ritual. Similar ritual mutilations are carried out by many savage tribes, but it is difficult to believe that a Stone Age man would have so handicapped himself in the struggle for existence. Great probability attaches to the suggestion that the pictures represent mutilations resulting from frost-bite or some other disease condition.

The performance of amputations by primitives is very rare, but the Masai of Africa did not hesitate to cut off a limb when it was absolutely necessary. A tight ligature was tied just above the line of amputation, the limb was placed on a hard, smooth log, and deftly chopped off by a single stroke of a sharp sword. There is some evidence that the Incas of Peru used to perform amputations, and North American Indians are said to have chopped off injured fingers. The latter operation was witnessed by the missionary William Ellis in the South Sea Islands. Ellis also reports the case of a native who operated on himself for femoral hernia, cutting away a portion of the intestine. Needless to say this attempt at do-it-yourself surgery ended fatally. According to the traveller A. H. Savage Landor, in Tibet, the lopping off of limbs for surgical reasons is undertaken but with fatal results. The necessity for amputation must always have existed, but most primitive peoples have a peculiar horror of such mutilating procedures—at least if carried out upon themselves. The cutting off of a hand or a foot was common enough as a punitive measure, but this cannot be regarded as surgery: neither can such procedures as scalping, tattooing, the production of tribal marks and scars, the perforation of the nose or the ears, the splitting of lips and similar ritual operations be considered as surgery in the strict sense of the word.

Another operation which may have originated in the prehistoric period is circumcision. Although it is generally believed that this operation was instituted by the Jews this is not the case. There is incontrovertible evidence, including pictorial and sculptured representations of the operation, that circumcision was carried out in ancient Egypt. It seems, however, that it was not practised on all males as is the case among the Jews and the Moslems. Certain carvings from Stone Age sites (Magdalenian period) in France show figures which seem to have undergone the operation of circumcision or some similar mutilation. This interpretation has not been generally accepted, but if it is correct it is by far the earliest record of the operation. Although there are hygienic reasons for carrying out this procedure there is little doubt that it originated as a religious rite. Other mutilating operations upon the genital

organs of both sexes have been carried out from time immemorial both by aboriginals and by so-called civilized peoples,
but these do not really come into the story of surgery.

The record of one major operation, a Caesarean section,
performed by a native operator in Uganda in 1879 has been
the subject of much debate and it is so extraordinary that until
quite recently medical historians were very doubtful about its
authenticity. The operation was witnessed by Robert W. Felkin,
a medical missionary, who described it in great detail and even
made sketches of what he saw. The patient was a young
woman of twenty years of age and it was her first pregnancy.
She was given plenty of banana wine and was tied to the bed.
The surgeon washed his hands and the patient's abdomen with
wine, then with water. After first pronouncing an incantation
he gave a shrill yell and then made a quick incision, cutting
through the abdomen and through the wall of the uterus.
Bleeding points were touched by an assistant with a red-hot
iron. The child was taken out quickly and handed over to an
assistant. The cord was cut and the after-birth was removed
by hand. The womb was not sutured, but the abdominal
wound was covered temporarily with a porous grass mat, and
the patient was raised to let the fluid out. Then the wound was
closed with seven thin nails and string, very much as a chicken
is trussed with skewers and string. The child was alive and the
mother made a perfect recovery, her wound being healed on
the eleventh day. There is now no doubt whatever as to the
authenticity of this case, and it may be mentioned that there
are several reliable records of women who have successfully
delivered themselves by Caesarean section. What is so very remarkable about the operation witnessed by Felkin is that the
patient was given banana wine as an analgesic, that antiseptic
precautions were taken, and that every step of the operation
was carefully planned in advance.

To sum up the surgical achievements of prehistoric and
primitive man, we find that the treatment of wounds in some
way or another is universal. There is great similarity between
the methods used in different parts of the world: the use of
naturally occurring styptic substances to control bleeding, the
application of powders and infusions with an astringent or

disinfectant action, protective bandaging, heat and massage. The results of wound treatment are often good—incomparably better than those seen in primitive treatment of internal ailments. The reasons for this, apart from the skilful methods which were often used, are the natural hardiness of the savage and the absence of the highly resistant germs encountered by civilized man.

The treatment of fractures and dislocations was generally rational, but the considerable skill shown in the application of splints is not always matched by equal care in reduction. Blood letting and the incision of boils and abscesses are commonly practised, but amputation and excision are very rarely performed. It may at first sight seem strange that the surgery of primitives, who show great manual skill and who carry out such major procedures as trephination of the skull, should otherwise be so limited in its scope. The main reason for this lack of advance is that the anatomical knowledge of primitive peoples is notoriously bad. Modern surgery rests upon the triple foundation of anatomy, anaesthesia, and asepsis. It is possible that some primitive peoples may have had means of producing both general and local anaesthesia, and although they knew nothing of asepsis their wound dressings often had an antiseptic action. Furthermore their constitutional resistance and the fact that they were generally treated in isolation enabled them to overcome wound infection relatively easily. Profound ignorance of body structure and function was the principal bar to any extension of surgery, and it was enhanced by the limiting influence of supernatural ideas. Surgery was not a special field of practice; the surgeon was the priest-physician or medicine-man. Only among the Masai, who are the master-surgeons of all native races, do we find a definite class of surgeons. Primitive surgery contains a large element of magic: the surgeon mutters incantations and charms are hung on the patient to ensure healing. But before smiling at the superstitious beliefs of our ancestors we should remember that the use of charms and talismans is widespread today and that there are still patients who refuse to undergo operations at times which the stars have declared to be unpropitious.

Not all the remarkable feats of native surgery recorded by

travellers and missionaries can be regarded as normal practice. Many of them probably represent unusual cases which have stood out in the memory. Nevertheless, primitive man had grasped the fundamental principles of wound treatment and he often showed remarkable ingenuity in devising instruments and appliances. Crude as his techniques may appear by modern standards, they represent landmarks in the evolution of surgery.

FOR FURTHER READING

Ackerknecht, E. H. Primitive surgery. *Amer. Anthrop.*, 1947, *49*, 25.

Black, W. G. *Folk Medicine.* 1883.

Brockbank, W. *Ancient Therapeutic Arts.* 1954.

Brodsky, I. The trephiners of Blanche Bay, New Britain. *Brit. J. Surg.*, 1938, *26*, 1.

Corlett, W. T. *The Medicine Man of the American Indians and his Cultural Background.* 1935.

Crump, J. A. Trephining in the South Seas. *J. Anthrop. Inst.*, 1901, *31*, 167.

Davies, J. N. P. The development of scientific medicine in the kingdom of Bunyoro-Kitara. *Med. Hist.*, 1959, *3*, 47.

Dawson, W. R. *Magician and Leech.* 1929.

Ford, E. Trephining in Melanesia. *Med. J. Australia*, 1937, ii, 471.

Harley, G. W. *Native African Medicine.* 1941.

Harvey, S. C. *The History of Hemostasis.* New York. 1929.

Hilton-Simpson, M. W. *Arab Medicine and Surgery: A Study of the Healing Art in Algeria.* 1922.

MacCurdy, G. G. Prehistoric surgery—a Neolithic Survival. *Amer. Anthrop.*, 1905, N.S. 7, 17.

Mackenzie, D. *The Infancy of Medicine.* 1927.

Moodie, R. L. *The Antiquity of Disease.* 1923.

Parry, T. W. The prehistoric trephined skulls of Great Britain. *Proc. Roy. Soc. Med. (Hist. Sect.)*, 1921, *14*, 27.

Sigerist, H. E. *A History of Medicine.* Vol. 1. 1951.

Stone, E. *Medicine among the American Indians.* 1932.

CHAPTER TWO

The Ancient East

OUR knowledge of prehistoric surgery is mainly conjectural, and although a good deal is known about the surgery of primitive peoples much remains to be discovered. In some respects we know more about the medicine and the surgery of the ancient civilizations—those of Sumer and Akkad, Babylonia, Assyria and Egypt, which flourished from about 4000 B.C. onwards—than we do about that of some primitive peoples still living in the world today. The existence of written records not only enables us to form a more exact idea of the surgical techniques which were followed but also to understand the ideas which lay behind them. Knowledge of primitive surgery often rests upon the unsupported testimony of early travellers who may not have grasped the exact significance of what they claim to have seen.

At the most remote period of recorded history the practice of medicine was still mainly magico-religious in character, but much of it was rational and there was a good deal of accumulated knowledge about disease. Thanks to the comparatively large number of documents that have survived and to the numerous objects that have been excavated from tombs and temples we know a good deal about the medicine and surgery of the ancient Egyptians. There are many gaps and some of the records are fragmentary, but enough survives to show that medicine was already becoming a science as well as an art. The ancient Egyptians enjoyed great fame as physicians. The Greek historian Herodotus, who visited Egypt in the fifth century B.C., was struck by the fact that there were so many specialists: "Medicine with them is distributed in the following way: every physician is for one disease and not for several, and the whole country is full of physicians; for there are physicians for the eyes, others for the head, others for the teeth, others for the belly, others for obscure diseases." The chief Egyptian physicians were attached to the Court and occupied positions of great honour and renown. One of them, Imhotep—the name means "He who cometh in Peace"—was vizier and physician to King Zoser who lived about 2980 B.C. Such was the fame of Imhotep that he was eventually raised to the status of a god and he became one of the principal Egyptian deities of healing. Physicians and surgeons (in spite of the high degree of specialization there was no clear-cut distinction between these two branches) were trained in temple schools and probably remained priests all their lives. There was a strong magical element in Egyptian medicine but religion overshadowed everything else. Almost every disease and every part of the body had its special god; some gods were the authors of disease while others gave protection against disease.

A number of Egyptian medical documents have survived in the form of papyrus rolls. The principal surviving texts range in date from about 2000 to 1200 B.C., but the knowledge and the ideas which they contain almost certainly relate to a considerably older period, perhaps five or six thousand years ago. The most interesting of the Egyptian papyri from the surgical point of view is the Edwin Smith Papyrus—so named from its discoverer, the American Egyptologist, Edwin Smith, who acquired it at Luxor in 1862. This work is a roll just over fifteen feet in length. It was composed at the beginning of the eighteenth dynasty, about 1600 B.C., and represents part of a large textbook of surgery. The surviving portion contains descriptions of forty-eight cases of injuries, wounds, fractures, dislocations, and tumours. The description of the cases follows the exact pattern of a modern textbook. The cases are listed in the order which has become traditional, namely, proceeding from the head to the feet. The surviving text breaks off abruptly in the middle of a discussion of the treatment of a spinal injury. What caused the scribe to interrupt his work in the middle of a sentence we shall never know, but it is a great pity that we do not possess the entire work. The unfinished portions would undoubtedly have dealt with injuries of the pelvis and lower extremities and it would have been interesting to know what the Egyptian surgeon had to say about abdominal diseases. Even in its fragmentary state the book is of extraordinary interest and importance because it is the oldest surgical work known and may in fact be the oldest "book" in the world.

The method of arrangement is first of all to set out the title or the chief symptom; then come the further symptoms, examination, diagnosis, prognosis and treatment. The advice given is entirely rational, as will be seen by the following directions for the treatment of a fractured humerus:

"Instructions concerning a break in his upper arm. If thou examinest a man having a break in his upper arm, and thou findest his upper arm hanging down, separated from its fellow, thou shouldst say concerning him: 'One having a break in his upper arm. An ailment which I will treat.'

"Thou shouldst place him prostrate on his back, with something folded between his two shoulder blades; thou shouldst spread out with his two shoulders in order to stretch apart his upper arm until that break falls into its place. Thou shouldst make for him two splints of linen, and thou shouldst apply for him one of them both on the inside of his arm, and the other of them both on the underside of his arm. Thou shouldst bind it with *ymrw* [an unidentified mineral substance], and treat it afterward with honey every day until he recovers."

This is how the Egyptian surgeon of nearly four thousand years ago treated a broken nose:

"If thou examinest a man having a break in the column of his nose, his nose being disfigured and a depression being in it, while the swelling there is on it protrudes, and he has discharged blood from both his nostrils, thou shouldst say concerning him: 'One having a break in the column of his nose. An ailment which I will treat.'

"Thou shouldst cleanse it with two plugs of linen. Thou shouldst place two other plugs of linen saturated with grease in the inside of his two nostrils. Thou shouldst (put him on his customary diet and administer no medicines) until the swelling is reduced. Thou shouldst apply for him stiff rolls of linen by which the nose is held fast. Thou shouldst treat him afterward with grease, honey and lint, every day until he recovers."

Trephination appears to have been very rarely practised in ancient Egypt, but in a case of depressed fracture of the skull the bony fragments were removed with an elevator. The edges of the wound were to be closely applied to each other and so bandaged. The Edwin Smith Papyrus contains the earliest known mention of the brain with its convolutions and meninges and there is little doubt that it was recognized as the seat of mental functions.

The following directions are given for the treatment of a wound in the forehead producing a compound comminuted fracture of the skull. In this serious case the ancient surgeon, for all his skill, feels compelled to invoke the aid of the gods.

"If thou examinest a man having a wound in his forehead, smashing the skull of his head. Thou shouldst prepare for him the egg of an ostrich, triturated with grease and placed in the mouth of his wound. Now afterward thou shouldst prepare for him the egg of an ostrich, triturated and made into poultices for drying up that wound. Thou shouldst apply to it for him a covering for the physician's use (i.e. a bandage); thou shouldst uncover it the third day, and find it knitting together the skull, the colour being like the egg of an ostrich.

"That which is to be said as a charm over this recipe:

"Repelled is the enemy that is in the wound!
Cast out is the evil that is in the blood.
The adversary of Horus, one every side of the mouth of
    Isis.
"This temple does not fall down;
There is no enemy of the vessel therein.
I am under the protection of Isis;
My rescue is the son of Osiris."

These are the directions for dealing with a gaping wound of the shoulder:

"If thou examinest a man having a gaping wound in his shoulder, its flesh being laid back and its sides separated, while he suffers with swelling in his shoulder blade, thou shouldst palpate his wound. Shouldst thou find its gash separated from its sides in his wound, as a roll of linen is unrolled, and it is painful when he raises his arm on account of it, thou shouldst draw together for him his gash with stitching. . . . Thou shouldst bind it with fresh meat the first day. If thou findest that wound open and its stitching loose, thou shouldst draw together for him its gash with two strips of linen over that gash; thou shouldst treat it afterward with grease, honey and lint every day until he recovers."

The application of fresh meat is prescribed in sixteen cases in the Edwin Smith Papyrus. This form of dressing still survives as a popular remedy; witness the raw steak treatment for a black eye. In ancient Egyptian practice meat was a preparatory remedy anticipating the application of other dressings such as grease and honey. Honey was often applied alone to a wound; in seventeen of the papyrus cases it was spread upon absorbent lint. This use of honey, incidentally, provides a striking example of the way in which ancient remedies are sometimes revived. In the 1930s—some 3,500 years after its use had been advocated by the physicians of Ancient Egypt—many German and Russian surgeons published articles on the value of honey as a wound dressing.

An interesting point in the case histories of the Edwin Smith papyrus is that after the diagnosis the writer gives a decision about his further course of action. The verdict takes one of three forms:

> An ailment which I will treat.
> An ailment with which I will contend.
> An ailment not to be treated.

This guarded attitude on the part of the medical man was widespread in antiquity. Whereas the present-day doctor does everything possible to alleviate symptoms to the very end even when the patient has no chance of recovery, the view in ancient times was that hopeless cases were not to be touched. The reasons for this are not far to seek. Those in attendance at the courts of ancient Egypt might expect rich rewards if their patient recovered, but if a patient died under their care the unfortunate physicians ran a grave risk of impalement.

It is quite clear from the evidence of the papyrus that the

ancient Egyptians were not without anatomical knowledge and that they had considerable experience of war surgery. They probed wounds, removed foreign bodies and pieces of broken bone, brought the edges of wounds together and either sutured them or kept them approximated by means of adhesive bandages, reduced fractures and dislocations, and had a variety of ointments, dressings, splints and instruments.

It is of interest to note that the Egyptian medical papyri contain far more evidence of magical practice, in the shape of charms and incantations, than do the surgical texts. The reason for this is that you cannot heal a broken leg or reduce a dislocated jaw with an incantation, but you can cure or improve a great many internal diseases by such means. That is, you can place the patient in a frame of mind that will reinforce the healing powers of nature. This fact was fully appreciated by the early physicians, many of whom were as skilled in the art—as opposed to the science—of medicine as their present-day counterparts.

Medicine also reached a high stage of development in ancient Babylon and Assyria. The seal of a Babylonian surgeon, Urlugaledin, dating from about 2300 B.C., is preserved in the Louvre. One of the earliest kings of Babylon, Hammurabi (1948–1905 B.C.), drew up a comprehensive code of laws which he caused to be engraved on a pillar of hard stone and set up in the temple. This celebrated Code of Hammurabi is also in the Louvre. The code contains laws relating to medical practice which show that medicine and surgery were highly organized professions. Fees were regulated and penalties were laid down for failure:

"Concerning the wounds resulting from operations it is written: if a physician shall produce on anyone a severe wound with a bronze operating knife and cure him, or if he shall open an abscess with the operating knife and preserve the eye of the patient, he usually shall receive 10 shekels of silver; if it is a slave, his master shall usually pay 2 shekels of silver to the physician.

"If a physician shall make a severe wound with an operating knife and kill him, or shall open an abscess with an operating knife and destroy the eye, his hands shall be cut off.

"If a physician shall make a severe wound with a bronze operating knife on the slave of a free man and kill him, he shall replace the slave with another slave. If he shall open an abscess with a bronze operating knife and destroy the eye, he shall pay the half of the value of the slave."

The Hammurabi Code also mentions the *Gallabu*, or barber-surgeons, whose province was minor surgery, including dentistry and the branding of slaves.

The library of Ashurbanipal, king of Assyria (668–626 B.C.) excavated by Sir Henry Layard at Nineveh, in 1845–6, is now in the British Museum. It consists of thirty thousand tablets of baked clay bearing cuneiform (wedge-shaped) writing. About eight hundred of these texts are medical. Some of the royal letters give us intimate glimpses of medical practice at this remote era: "Now the handmaid of the king, Bau-Gamelat, is seriously ill, she does not eat a morsel. Now may the king my lord give instructions: may a physician come to see her." A letter addressed to king Esarhaddon refers to the extraction of teeth: "Replying to what the king my lord wrote me, 'Send me your true diagnosis.' I have given my diagnosis to the king, my lord, in one word: 'Inflammation.' He whose head, hands and feet are inflamed owes his state to his teeth: his teeth shall be extracted. On this account his insides are inflamed. The pain will presently subside, the condition will be most satisfactory."

Surgical instruments of bronze were also found at Nineveh, and in this respect the Assyrians may not have been so well equipped as the Egyptians. Iron was used in Egypt as early as 1600 B.C. There is great similarity between the Egyptian and the Assyrian medical texts, both being strange medleys of rational therapy with magical spells and incantations According to the testimony of Herodotus, Babylonian medicine must have declined in the fifth century B.C. He states that there were no physicians, but that the people brought their sick into the market-place in order that passers-by might make suggestions or pass on cures.

The medical history of India is extremely interesting but its records contain much legendary lore. The earliest texts, which date from about 1500 B.C., show that treatment of diseases at that time consisted mainly of spells and incantations, but by the fifth century B.C. a more or less rational system of medicine had evolved. In certain fields the medicine of the ancient Hindus takes priority over that of the Greeks. Operations, such as that for anal fistula, are described in the Indian texts which are not mentioned in the writings of Hippocrates. This is also true of the plastic operations which are characteristic of Indian medicine and which did not come into use in the rest of the world until the late medieval period.

The two greatest figures in the medical history of India are Charaka, who lived at the beginning of the Christian era and wrote mainly on internal diseases, and Susruta, of the fifth century A.D., whose writings deal with surgery. Susruta is supposed to have learned his art as a pupil of Dhanvantari, the physician of the gods. The qualifications and equipment of the surgeons as set down by Susruta are practically the same as would be recommended at the present day. He advocated the dissection of dead bodies as indispensable for a student, and gives detailed advice on the acquisition of the manual skills which are necessary for the surgeon. The art of making specific incisions should be taught by cutting into the body of a gourd, water melon, or cucumber. The student should be trained to cut either in an upward or downward direction and with either hand. Excisions and evacuations should be demonstrated by taking seeds out of fruit, by making openings in the body of a full water-bag, the bladder of a dead animal, or in the side of a leather pouch full of water or slime. Seeds should be extracted from fruits and pith from the stems of plants. Bandaging was to be practised on full-sized manikins made of stuffed linen.

Susruta describes a great variety of surgical instruments, including knives, cauteries, saws, syringes, scissors, hooks, forceps, trocars, catheters, specula, sounds, and needles for suturing. Exact directions are given for the incision of abscesses in various parts of the body. After the operation the patient should be washed with hot water, the abscess should be pressed with the fingers for complete evacuation, then washed with an astringent solution. Into the opening of the abscess a strip of cloth impregnated with sesame and honey was inserted, after which the abscess was covered first with a poultice, then with a cloth neither too thick nor too thin, and bound. On the third day the bandage was removed and renewed.

The list of surgical operations given by Susruta shows that the Hindus knew the operations for anal fistula, tonsillectomy, and Caesarean section. Blood vessels were ligated with the fibres of plants, but the cautery, boiling oil and pressure were also used for checking haemorrhage. Four kinds of sutures are described—hemp, flax, bark fibre, and hair; and three kinds of needles—round, triangular and curved. The treatment of fractures and dislocations is described with great accuracy. Limbs were amputated and iron substitutes provided. Stone in the bladder is also exactly described and minute directions are given for operation, which was regarded as necessary when medical treatment had failed. The technique of operation was the same as that used in Europe up to the end of the sixteenth century. The patient was placed with his legs spread apart and tied down separately. The incision was made over the stone in the left part of the perineum, and about two fingers' breadth from the anus. The opening was then enlarged according to the size of the stone which was removed with iron forceps. Care had to be taken not to break the stone or to leave fragments inside the body. The importance of avoiding injury to the seminal vessels, the spermatic cord and the rectum was also stressed. Great attention was paid to post-operative care.

There are also directions for the operation on tumours of the neck, for incision in cases of dropsy, for removal of the tonsils, which is done with a semi-circular knife after the tonsils have been seized with forceps and drawn downwards. Advice is given for the treatment of prolapse of the rectum.

The great highlight of Hindu surgery was, however, the operation of rhinoplasty—the making of a new nose. This procedure was in some demand owing to the fact that adulterers were punished by having their noses cut off. The operation appears to have been carried out mainly by members of the caste of the potters, among whom it was an hereditary skill.

As described by Susruta the procedure was as follows:

"First the leaf of a creeper, long and broad enough to fully cover the whole of the severed or clipped off part, should be gathered, and a patch of loving flesh, equal in dimensions to the preceding leaf, should be sliced off (from down upward) from the cheek and after scarifying it with a knife, swiftly adhered to the severed nose. Then the cool-headed physician should steadily tie it up with a bandage decent to look at and perfectly suited to the end for which it has been employed. The physician should make sure that the adhesion of the severed parts has been fully effected and then insert two small pipes into the nostrils to facilitate respiration, and to prevent the adhesioned flesh from hanging down after that, the adhesioned part should be dusted with the powders of Pattanga, Yashtimadhukam and Rasanjana pulverized together; and the nose should be enveloped in Karpasa cotton and several times sprinkled over with the refined oil or pure sesamum. . . . Adhesion should be deemed complete after the incidental ulcer had been perfectly healed up, while the nose should be again scarified and bandaged in the case of a semi or partial adhesion. The adhesioned nose should be tried to be elongated where it would fall short of its natural and previous length, or it should be surgically restored to its natural size in the case of the abnormal growth of its newly formed flesh."

A similar technique was used in making a new lobe of the ear and in repairing a severed lip. Another method of nose repair, by taking a flap from the forehead, was practised in India from time immemorial. This technique was re-discovered at the beginning of the nineteenth century by the English surgeon Joseph Constantine Carpue, as will be described later (page 135).

Susruta also describes the treatment of perforating wounds of the abdomen. In a case of protrusion of the intestines they should be carefully examined, washed with milk, lubricated with clarified butter, and gently re-introduced into their natural position. If the intestine itself is perforated the tear should be closed by applying black ants—the method which has already been mentioned as forming part of the surgical practice of several primitive peoples. Intestinal obstruction is to be treated by incision, extraction of any concretion or foreign body, replacement of the parts after moistening them with honey and butter, and sewing up of the incision.

There is no doubt that most of the surgical procedures described by Susruta were actually carried out by him, but some of the anecdotes which he relates concerning the practice of other surgeons strain our credulity. A good example is the case of a Rajah who was suffering from excruciating pain in the head. All the ordinary methods of treatment had been tried but in vain and his condition was critical, when two strangers arrived at the court and it was learned that they were physicians. Called into consultation, they held that unless surgically treated the royal patient could obtain no relief. "Accordingly they administered an anaesthetic called *Sammohini* with a view to render him insensible and, when completely under the influence of the drug, they trephined his skull, removing the malignant portion of the brain, the actual seat of the complaint, closed and stitched up the opening, and applied healing balm to the wound. They then administered a restorative known as *Sanjivani* to the patient, who, thereupon, regained consciousness and felt quite at ease."

An even more wonderful story is recorded of King Buddhadisa of Ceylon, who lived in the fourth century A.D. This good monarch was a patron of learning and a pioneer of social medicine. He not only established hospitals and appointed physicians for all the villages in his kingdom, but was accustomed to carry a case of surgical instruments with him and to proffer help to every afflicted person that he met. His most notable case was that of the herdsman who drank some water very quickly. "The water contained frogs' eggs, and one of these, entering a nostril, continued onward into the head. Within the skull the egg developed and a frog came forth, so that in rainy weather he would croak and gnaw the head of the herdsman. The Rajah split the head of the man and removed the frog, after which he brought the incised parts together and the wound healed very quickly."

The reputed father of Chinese medicine was the Emperor Shen Nung who lived about 3000 B.C. He discovered a large number of remedies and poisons which he described in the *Pen Tsao* or Great Herbal which contains particulars of over a thousand drugs. Chinese medicine, like that of other early civilizations, gradually escaped from the control of magic and sorcery. Complicated theories were evolved, the most important of which was that of the two vital principles or life forces— Yang (masculine)and Yin (feminine). These two principles or opposing qualities governed all the bodily functions and the chief cause of all diseases was thought to be some disturbance of their balance or an arrest of their flow.

The principal means adopted to restore the balance of the "humours" in case of illness was counter-irritation by acupuncture. Acupuncture, which is said to have been practised from about 2700 B.C., consisted in the introduction of long, fine needles into the body at various specified points. The aim was to penetrate one or more of the canals which were supposed to carry the two vital principles to the organs. This was thought to remove obstructions and allow the escape of bad secretions. The needles were made of gold, silver, steel or iron and were one to ten inches in length. They were sometimes heated. This counter-irritation method still survives and actually enjoys considerable vogue in France at the present day. Acupuncture was often accompanied by the application of moxa, that is, burning on the skin the powdered leaves of mugwort (*Artemesia vulgaris*) to which a little incense was added. These forms of treatment were widespread throughout the Far East. The craze for acupuncture is a comparatively modern one in the West, but moxa was used by European surgeons in a number of conditions up to the end of the eighteenth century.

According to Chinese annals, Yu Fu, a surgeon who lived in the reign of Huang Ti, the Yellow Emperor (2698–2598 B.C.), made incisions through the skin, dissected the muscles, tied blood vessels, sutured tendons, exposed the brain and spinal cord, and cleansed the stomach and intestines. In the time of the Tsin dynasty there was a surgeon, a pupil of Yin Chung-k'an, who did plastic surgery for harelip. His patients were required to live on a liquid diet for a hundred days and to abstain from laughter. Another surgeon, Fang Kan, who lived in the T'ang dynasty, was so proficient in this department of surgery that he was called "The Doctor of Lips' Repair". In the Chou dynasty Pien Ch'iao operated on the heart and the stomach.

Castration—an operation very common in the ancient world—is mentioned in Chinese records dating from before 1000 B.C., and was performed by specialists in order to produce eunuchs for the Imperial Court. It seems that some form of general or local anaesthesia was used, and that the organs were amputated with a semi-circular knife. An astringent powder composed of alum and various resins was applied to the wound and pressure was exerted until the haemorrhage stopped. Then a wood or metal catheter was introduced into the urethra. Healing generally took place after the third month. Mortality was probably very high, but the estimates vary greatly—between two and fifty per cent. The excised parts were preserved in alcohol so that they could be buried with the body after death, because according to Chinese religious beliefs it is not possible for a dead person with a mutilated body to be reunited with his ancestors. This barbarous mutilation was still carried out at the Imperial Court at the end of the nineteenth century, and according to reliable witnesses the method of anaesthesia then practised was to knock the patient out by a sudden blow on the jaw.

The most famous surgeon of China is Hua To (A.D. 115–205). His exploits became legendary and he was, in fact, often worshipped as the God of Surgery. As a young man he was roaming over the hills when he came across two sages in a grotto. The wise men were so impressed by his conversation that they gave him a book containing all the secrets of medicine. When Hua To had mastered the contents of this invaluable work he embarked on his career as a physician and surgeon. He used few drugs, but was a pioneer of hydrotherapy. He is said to have cured a woman patient of a long continued fever by seating her inside a stone trough and ordering his assistants to pour one hundred bucketsful of cold water over her.

Hua To is also generally reputed to have been the discoverer of surgical anaesthesia, although some say that Pien Ch'iao had used anaesthetics four hundred years earlier. Hua To made his patients take an effervescing powder in wine which produced numbness and insensibility. He is said to have opened the abdomen and to have washed out or removed diseased parts. After suturing, he applied special salves which brought about healing within a few days and his patients were able to resume all their normal activities within a month. Hua To is also reputed to have carried out a successful removal of the spleen—an operation that was not performed in Europe until the nineteenth century and which is still regarded as a formidable undertaking. A long list of this great surgeon's remarkable cures is given by the Chinese annalists, and there is no mention of failures! Hua To sometimes worked without an anaesthetic, as in the case of Kuan Kung, a famous general of the Three Kingdoms, upon whom he operated for a poisoned arrow wound of the arm. To detract the patient's attention from the painful manipulations a game of chess was played.

In the Wei dynasty (A.D. 225) there is record of a Caesarean section being performed upon the wife of a Tartar prince. Both mother and child survived. Chinese surgery made no progress after the Tang dynasty (A.D. 619–907) and no books were written on the subject. In spite of the achievements of Hua To and other operators, the Chinese surgeon has always occupied a position inferior to that of the physician.

Chinese medicine was introduced into Japan by way of Korea. The earliest Japanese surgical books were written in the ninth centry A.D. and were based on Chinese models. The *Ishinho*, of Yasuhori Tamba (A.D. 892), describes various surgical procedures such as the opening of abscesses, the application of the cautery to ulcers and to bites of mad dogs, and the stitching of wounds of the intestine with threads made of the fibre of the mulberry tree. Inflammations were treated by the application of leeches, cold stones or iron, or white of egg. Cataract was treated by "needling". Much was learned from contact with Dutch and other foreign doctors from the sixteenth century onwards, and a number of standard European textbooks were translated into Japanese. Seishu Hanoaka (1760–1833) was the first Japanese surgeon to amputate limbs, to extirpate tumours, and to operate for cancer of the tongue and for anal fistula. He is said to have administered a narcotic, an infusion of aconite, datura and other plants, before operating.

The Bible contains many references to diseases, especially to plague and other epidemics, but tells us very little about surgery apart from simple wound treatment. The Hebrews regarded disease as a visitation from God and as providing little scope for human intervention. One direction in which they were definite pioneers was in the field of public health. The Old Testament has many references to the importance of personal hygiene, and Moses has been regarded as the author of the first sanitary code.

Circumcision—the one operation that was universally practised—did not originate with the Jews. In early times it was carried out with a sharp stone, and the practice continued even when bronze instruments were in use because the forms of the ancient rite were preserved.

The Talmud, that great repository of traditional Jewish law which originated between the second and the sixth centuries, contains some interesting anatomical and physiological data but not very much that is relevant to surgery. Among the surgical instruments mentioned are the large and small knife, cupping-glasses, trephine and lancet. The surgeon was advised to wear a leather apron when operating, and he was warned not to allow his hands to touch the wound because "the hand causes inflammation"—an interesting anticipation of modern ideas regarding the transmission of infection. For severe operations the patient was given a preliminary sleeping draught. Wounds and ulcers were treated with oil and warm water, balsam, and compresses of vinegar and wine. Poisoned wounds were sucked and in some cases cauterized with hot irons. Blood letting was a favourite method of treatment and was carried out by incision or by leeches. There is also mention of Caesarean section, amputation, trephination, an operation for the removal of excessive fat, and one for the formation of an artificial anus in cases of stricture. All these procedures are, however, dealt with from the legal and ritualistic points of view rather than the surgical, and we are left in doubt as to the extent to which they were actually performed by the Jewish physicians of this period.

FOR FURTHER READING

Breasted, J. H. *The Edwin Smith Surgical Papyrus*. 2 vols. Chicago. 1930.

Brim, C. J. *Medicine in the Bible*. New York. 1936.

Conteneau, G. *La Médecine en Assyrie et en Babylonie*. Paris. 1938.

Fujikawa, Y. *Japanese Medicine* (Clio Medica). New York. 1934.

Gondal, Maharajah of. *A Short History of Aryan Medical Science*. Gondal. 1890.

Hurry, J. B. *Imhotep, the Vizier and Physician of King Zoser and afterwards the Egyptian God of Medicine*. 2nd ed. 1928.

Leake, C. D. *The Old Egyptian Medical Papyri*. Lawrence, Kansas. 1952.

Morse, W. R. *Chinese Medicine* (Clio Medica). New York, 1934.

Mukhopadhyaya, G. *The Surgical Instruments of the Hindus*. 2 vols. Calcutta. 1913–14.

Snowman, J. *A Short History of Talmudic Medicine*. 1935.

Susruta. *An English Translation of the Sushruta Samhita*. By K. K. L. Bhishagratna. 2 vols. Calcutta. 1907–16.

Thompson, R. C. Assyrian medical texts. *Proc. Roy. Soc. Med.* (*Hist. Sect.*), 1924, *17*, 1; 1926, *19*, 29.

Wong, K.C. and Wu Lien-Teh. *History of Chinese Medicine*. 2nd ed. Shanghai. 1936.

Zimmer, H. R. *Hindu Medicine*. 1948.

CHAPTER THREE

Greeks and Romans

THE Greeks were the first people to separate medicine from magic and to base their practice upon observation and investigation; but this did not come about until a relatively late period in Greek history. Medicine may have reached a high level in the Minoan civilization of Crete which flourished from the fourth to the second millennium B.C., but we have no direct evidence of this. Many documents have been found in the course of excavations in Crete and, thanks to the remarkable progress that has been made recently in the decipherment of the peculiar Minoan script, we may soon know more about the medicine and surgery of this era. The ancient Egyptian medical books attribute prescriptions to the Cretan physicians, who already held a high reputation. But if the Egyptians borrowed from the pre-Hellenic Greeks, the Greeks in turn borrowed from their neighbours. All the knowledge of the ancient civilizations of the Near East came to Greece, where it was studied critically and transmuted by the Greek genius.

The early history of Greek medicine is very obscure, the only literary evidence we have being the poems of Homer. Here everything is overlaid by myth and legend, but nevertheless the poet provides us with an unforgettable picture of surgery at the time of the Trojan war. The *Iliad* and the *Odyssey* contain realistic descriptions of 140 wounds and injuries of widely differing types and, according to a German scholar who has investigated the point, they carried an overall mortality rate of 77.6 per cent. The most dangerous wounds were sword and spear thrusts and the least dangerous those inflicted by arrows. Everyone seemed able to do front-line surgery. Thus we read in the *Iliad* of Eurypylus having his thigh transfixed by an arrow and being succoured by his friend Patroclus:

"Patroclus, with his dagger, from the thigh
Cut out the biting shaft; and from the wound
With tepid water cleans'd the clotted blood;
Then pounded in his hands, a root applied
Astringent, anodyne, which all his pain
Allay'd; the wound was dried, and stanch'd with blood."

And in the *Odyssey* when Ulysses is gored by a wild boar, which tears the sinews and bares the bone:

"With bandage firm Ulysses' knee they bound;
Then, chanting mystic lays, the closing wound
Of sacred melody confessed the force:
The tides of life regained their azure course."

Here we have a typical example of the mixture of rational and irrational elements in early surgery—the firm bandage and the "mystic lays". But perhaps we should not thus lightly dismiss the healing power of music: some present-day American surgeons habitually operate to the strains of soothing melodies.

Apart from the amateur surgeons, the Greek expeditionary force was also supplied with professional healers skilled in the extraction of embedded weapons, the arrest of haemorrhage, and the alleviation of pain. Chief of these were the two sons of Aesculapius, Podalirius and Machaon. When Machaon's shoulder is pierced by an arrow, he is quickly carried from the fight in Nestor's chariot, for:

"A wise physician skilled our wounds to heal
Is more than armies to the public weal."

The combination of magico-religious rites with simple rational therapy is also seen in the Greek cult of "Incubation" or "Temple Sleep". Incubation was practised as early as the fourth century B.C. and it continued into the Christian era. The ritual was carried out in the Asklepieia or temples of Aesculapius, the Greek god of medicine. These temples were situated in places noted for their pure air and scenic beauty, and sick people resorted to them in large numbers. Sacrifices were made, the patient was bathed, and he then lay down to sleep in the colonnade of the temple. The god appeared to the patient in a dream and gave advice or in certain cases performed an operation. Tame snakes assisted in the treatment by licking the eyes and the sores of the patient. In the morning the patient departed cured. Tablets recording the cures (but not the failures) were set up in the temple, and the grateful patient presented a "votive offering", which took the form of a clay or stone model of the diseased part. Thus a patient who had suffered from varicose veins would give a realistic model of the affected limb. Many votive offerings in the shape of eyes, ears, arms, legs, breasts, and other parts of the body have survived from this period and may be seen in museums. In time physical therapy, diet, bathing and exercise came to play an increasingly important part in the temple cures and the routine was much the same as would be followed at a modern spa.

The first great step in the separation of the art of healing from superstition and magic was taken by Hippocrates, the "Father of Medicine", in the fifth century B.C. Hippocrates led a wandering life, practising and teaching in various parts of Greece, and he recorded his observations in writing. His accounts of actual cases are model clinical records and many of his descriptions of diseases could, with very few changes, take their place in a modern textbook. Not all the writings which go under the name of Hippocrates represent the sole work of the master himself; many of them were no doubt written by his pupils, but all bear the mark of his inspiration.

Hippocrates treated every kind of malady and his writings deal with many surgical disorders. He had great faith in the healing power of nature and favoured the use of simple dressings. He used tepid or cold water, with or without vinegar, wine, oil and honey. He knew that dry wounds were better than wet ones and that greasy dressings should be avoided. The edges of clean wounds were kept as closely approximated as possible and healing by first intention sometimes took place. He lays down rules for the arrangement of the surgery and describes many instruments. Surgeons then, as now, were liable to be called out at any hour of the day or night, hence the advice: "Have also another apparatus ready to hand for journeys, simply prepared, and handy too by method of arrangement, for one cannot overhaul everything."

Scalpels of different shapes seem to have been carried in boxes, probably wooden, which opened in two halves like a modern mathematical instrument box. In these the scalpels lay head and tail, separated from each other by small fixed partitions. Probes and forceps were carried in cylindrical cases like those in which scribes carried their pens. Many portable outfits of this type have been found with Roman remains, also boxes for medicines, divided into little compartments.

The Hippocratic treatise on fractures and dislocations is based on long experience and an accurate knowledge of the anatomy and physiology of bones and joints. Simple and compound fractures are distinguished and the process of bone repair by the formation of callus is described. Detailed instructions are given for reduction, bandaging, and immobilization of the limbs. Dislocation of the humerus was reduced with the aid of an assistant by placing the foot in the armpit or by manipulation with the arm hanging over a ladder or branch. For a dislocated femur a wooden apparatus resembling a rack was used. The principles of extension and counter-extension were fully understood. Important directions were given for reduction of dislocations of the shoulder, hands, fingers and jaw. In certain cases of jaw fracture the teeth were bound together with gold wire.

Injuries of the head are described in detail. Trephination of the skull should be performed in such a way that the instrument does not penetrate quickly to the dura mater. The trephine should be plunged frequently into cold water to avoid over-heating of the bone. Rectal disorders were diagnosed with the aid of the speculum. Piles were treated with suppositories, with the cautery, or finally by excision.

Hippocrates was on the whole against the incision of varicose veins, but in some cases he advocated puncture of the varix in as many places as possible. The earliest record of a surgical operation for varicose veins is in the case of the Roman consul Marius (155–86 B.C.). This case record is preserved for us in Plutarch's *Lives*:

"Marius, Roman consul and general, is praised for both temperance and endurance, of which latter he gave a decided instance in an operation of surgery. For having, as it seems, both his legs full of great tumours, and disliking the deformity, he determined to put himself into the hands of an operator; when, without being tied, he put out one of his legs, and silently, without changing countenance, endured a most excessive torment in the cutting, never flinching or complaining; but when the surgeon went to the other, he declined to have it done, saying, 'I see the cure is not worth the pain.' "

The Hippocratic surgeons were also expert in the treatment of disorders of the eye, ear, nose and throat, and the teeth. Operations were not, however, embarked upon lightly, and great reliance was placed upon diet, gymnastics, exercise, massage and sea-bathing.

Following the conquests of Alexander the Great, Greek culture came into close contact with the ancient culture of the Orient. Alexandria, founded in 332 B.C., became a great cosmopolitan centre of learning and the home of a notable medical school. Unfortunately, no surgical writings have come down to us from the Alexandrian school but from later records we know that great advances were made. These advances were mainly due to the work of two men, Herophilus and Erasistratus, both of whom flourished from the end of the fourth to the middle of the third century B.C. Herophilus may have been the first to practise public dissection of the human body, and he made very important contributions to anatomy. Erasistratus is often regarded as the founder of physiology. These two distinguished investigators have been accused of practising human vivisection upon criminals, but there is no conclusive evidence of this.

The golden age of Greek surgery was the first century A.D., when the advances in anatomical and physiological knowledge had been assimilated and had led to improved techniques for the performance of a number of operations.

An excellent account of surgical practice at this time is given in the encyclopaedic work of Celsus. This work was written in Latin about A.D. 30 and is one of the greatest monuments of Graeco-Roman medicine. Roman medicine hardly existed as a separate entity. The practice of medicine was beneath the dignity of a Roman citizen and most of the medical and surgical practice of Rome was in the hands of Greeks. Many of these practitioners were slaves in Roman families. Celsus was one of the very few Roman writers on medicine.

According to Celsus, the surgeon "should be youthful or in early middle age, with a strong and steady hand, as expert with the left hand as with the right, with vision sharp and clear, and spirit undaunted; so far void of pity that while he wishes only to cure his patient, yet is not moved by his cries to go too fast, or cut less than is necessary". Many surgical instruments of the time of Celsus were found in the ruins of Pompeii (destroyed A.D. 79) and these can be seen in the museum at Naples.

The surgery of Celsus shows a notable advance over that of the time of Hippocrates. Celsus first described the four cardinal signs of inflammation—heat, pain, redness and swelling—which are still learned by every medical student. To these signs Galen added a fifth—loss of function. Celsus deals with the complications that may follow wounds, including erysipelas and gangrene. He recommends that an injured vessel should be tied in two places and divided between them, but it is his younger contemporary, the surgeon Heliodorus, who gives the first account of terminal ligature and of torsion. Speaking of the operation for hernia he says, "We ligature the larger vessels, but as for the smaller ones, we catch them with hooks, and twist them many times, thus closing their mouths." For head wounds trephination is recommended and for dropsy puncture of the abdomen and drainage. For abdominal injuries the large intestine was sutured when damaged, but according to Celsus, there was no hope of curing wounds of the small intestine. Excision was recommended for cancer of the breast but only when it was diagnosed early. Several eye operations are described including couching for cataract. This latter procedure was accomplished with a needle which is "inserted through the two coats of the eye until it meets resistance, and then the cataract is pressed down so that it may settle in the lower part." Tonsillectomy as described by Celsus is the modern method of enucleation. Plastic surgery occupies an important place, especially that of the nose and other parts of the head, and Celsus outlines methods of repair by using the skin of neighbouring parts. Bladder surgery had made considerable progress and there are exact directions for removing and for crushing stones.

The early Greek surgeons were very loath to perform amputations. Hippocrates does not mention amputation in the strict sense but only the removal of the dead part in case of gangrene of a limb. Celsus still describes amputation as "the last sad remedy", but some of his contemporaries and immediate successors certainly carried out amputations by essentially modern methods. In the hands of Archigenes (end of first century A.D.) the operation assumes quite a modern shape. The indications for amputation include not only gangrene but chronic ulcers, malignant tumours, severe injury and great deformity. In some cases the whole part to be removed should be sprinkled with cold water and bandaged, the limb being then tightly constricted with a cord above the point of amputation; where this is not practicable the chief arteries going to the part should be cut down upon and tied.

The surgeons of the Roman Empire seem to have been acquainted with amputation by flaps as well as with the circular method. Thus Heliodorus writes: "Amputation above the elbow or knee is very dangerous owing to the size of the vessels divided. Some operators in their foolish haste cut through all the soft parts at one stroke, but it seems to me better to first divide the flesh on the side away from the vessels, and then to saw the bone, so as to be ready at once to check the bleeding when the large vessels are cut. And before operating I am wont to tie a ligature as tightly as possible above the point of amputation." The flap operation is still more clearly described in his directions for removing a supernumerary finger. "A circular incision is made round the digit near its base. From this two vertical incisions are made opposite one another and the flaps so formed dissected up. The base being thus laid bare the digit is to be removed by cutting forceps and the flaps are then brought together and sutured."

The ancients were very skilful in the use of probes or sounds. This is how Celsus describes the examination of a fistula: "But first it is well to put a probe into the fistula to learn where it goes and how deeply it reaches, also whether it is moist or rather dry as is evident when the probe is withdrawn. Further, if there be bone adjacent, it is possible to learn whether the fistula has entered it or not and how deeply it has caused disease. For if the part is soft which is reached by the end of the probe the disease is still intermuscular; if the resistance be greater it has reached the bone; if there the probe slips there is as yet no caries. If it does not slip but meets with a uniform resistance there is indeed caries, but it is as yet slight. If what is below is uneven and rough the bone is seriously eroded, and whether there is cartilage below will be known by the situation, and if the disease has reached it, will be evident from the resistance." This passage is very significant. It shows that the surgeon of nearly two thousand years ago tried to arrive at an exact diagnosis before embarking on treatment. The history of the illness and of the patient's symptoms, careful physical examination, and assessment of the probabilities on the basis of the doctor's findings and of his past experience: this is the method of Hippocrates; and it is what distinguishes scientific medicine from primitive medicine and from quackery.

Celsus says sutures should be of soft thread, not over-twisted, that they may be the more easy on the part. They were commonly made of flax but Galen also refers to sutures of wool. There is no mention of catgut being used for surgical purposes although it is known that the Greek harp was strung with that substance. Wounds were also closed by fibulae or small metal clasps. The cautery was employed not only to control bleeding but as a counter-irritant, as a cutting instrument, and as a means of destroying tumours.

The greatest name in ancient medicine after Hippocrates is that of Galen, who was born at Pergamum in Asia Minor in A.D. 130. He had the largest practice in Rome and was physician successively to the emperors Marcus Aurelius, Commodus, and Septimus Severus. Galen was primarily a physician and an experimental physiologist, but before coming to Rome he had held the post of surgeon to the gladiators of his native city. This must have provided him with plenty of experience of wounds and injuries and his voluminous writings contain much about surgery. Galen describes some operations not previously recorded, such as resection of a rib to facilitate removal of pus from the chest and resection of the sternum with exposure of the heart. Galen gives careful directions for the treatment of wounds and pays attention to the general condition of the patient. He advocated conservative resection rather than amputation, and altogether his surgical writings provide evidence of considerable advance.

The name of Antyllus (second century A.D.) is connected with the earliest operation for aneurysm. He described two varieties of aneurysm: those that proceed from a local dilatation of the artery and are in a cylindrical form, and those that come from a lesion of the vessel and are rounded. Some aneurysms Antyllus would not treat because of the volume of the vessels and the danger of isolating and tying them, but in those situated upon the extremities and the head he operated in the following manner:

"If the aneurysm be by dilatation, make a straight incision through the skin in the direction of the length of the vessel, and, drawing open by the aid of hooks the lips of the wound, divide with precautions the membranes which cover the artery. With blunt hooks we isolate the vein from the artery, and lay bare on all sides the dilated part of this last vessel. After having introduced beneath the artery a probe, we raise the tumour and pass along the probe a needle armed with a double thread in such a manner that this thread finds itself placed beneath the artery; cut the threads near the extremity of the needle, so that there will be two threads having four ends; seizing, then, the two ends of one of these threads we bring it gently toward one of the two extremities of the aneurysm, tying it carefully; in like manner also we bring the other thread toward the opposite extremity, and in this place tie the artery. Thus the whole aneurysm is between the two ligatures. We open then the middle of the tumour by a small incision: in this manner all which it contains will be evacuated, and there will be no danger of haemorrhage."

Cataract received much attention from the Greek surgical

masters and they described four methods of removing the opaque lens:

(1) the cataract may be simply depressed or "couched".
(2) it may be extracted entire, a method first mentioned by Galen as a recent invention.
(3) the lens may be broken up and left to be absorbed.
(4) the lens may be broken up and at once removed by suction.

As already mentioned, the Romans despised medicine as a profession but this did not prevent them from making use of Greek physicians or even of the services of their own slaves. Galen tells us that in his time large cities such as Rome and Alexandria swarmed with specialists, who also travelled about from place to place. Martial mentions some of them in an epigram: "Cascellius extracts and repairs bad teeth; you, Hyginus, cauterize ingrowing eyelashes; Fannius cures a relaxed uvula without cutting; Eros removes brand marks from slaves; Hermes is a very Podalirius for ruptures." In Republican Rome military service was the privilege of every citizen and there is no mention of army surgeons. The soldiers seem to have carried bandages and perhaps other appliances with them and no doubt acquired some rude surgical skill. Under the Empire military medicine was highly organized: every cohort had its surgeon, and surgeons of a higher grade were attached to the legions as consultants. Army surgeons ranked as noncombatants and enjoyed many privileges. Memorial inscriptions to medical officers dying on service have been found in many countries, including Britain. The Emperor Trajan personally treated the wounded and when bandages gave out cut his own clothing into strips to bind the wounds of his soldiers. Military hospitals were maintained throughout the provinces, and this was long before there were any general hospitals open to all kinds of patients.

After the fall of the Roman Empire in the West medicine was kept alive by a number of learned physicians of Byzantium (Constantinople). Oribasius (A.D. 325–403), physician to the Emperor Julian, wrote a work on medicine and surgery in seventy books, of which twenty-five remain. Another Byzantine writer, Aetius of Amida (early sixth century) studied at Alexandria and practised in Byzantium in the time of the Emperor Justinian. He gives excellent descriptions of diseases of the ear, nose and throat and of goitre, hydrophobia, urethral disorders and haemorrhoids. The writings of Aetius and his contemporaries show evidence of the influence of the strong religious feeling of the age. Thus, in his directions for removing a bone from the throat, Aetius says it may be extracted by forceps or the patient may be given a piece of raw meat on a string which is to be pulled up when he has swallowed it; but the operator is also to say, "Bone come forth, like as Christ brought Lazarus from the tomb and Jonah from the whale." Alexander of Tralles, a younger contemporary of Aetius, includes with his medical advice a number of charms and absurd prescriptions, such as, "Take a live dung beetle, put him in a red rag, and hang him down the patient's neck."

Paul of Aegina (seventh century), the last of the great Byzantine medical writers, made few original contributions to surgery, but his writings provide a very complete picture of the surgical practice of his age. The operations of lithotomy, trephination, tonsillectomy, abdominal incision, and amputation of the breast are described in much greater detail than by any of his predecessors. According to Paul the most frequent sites of cancer are the uterus and the breast. He regarded operation on the former as useless in view of the rapidity of recurrence, but taught that some breast cancers could be extirpated. He condemned the use of the cautery in cases of cancer, but recommended it for various internal conditions such as abscess of the liver and diseases of the spleen. That removal of the tonsils was a standard procedure at this time is shown by the fact that special scalpels with opposite curvatures were designed for removal of the right or left tonsil. This is how Paul describes the operation: "Wherefore, having seated the patient in the sunlight, and directed him to open his mouth, one assistant holds his head and another presses down the tongue with a tongue depressor. We take a hook and perforate the tonsil with it and drag it outwards as much as we can without dragging the capsule out along with it, and then we cut it off by the root with the tonsillotome suited to that hand, for there are two such instruments having opposite curvatures. After the excision of one we may operate on the other in the same way."

In summing up the surgical achievements of the Greeks and Romans, it cannot be said that they introduced many new operations; most of the procedures carried out by them were known to the surgeons of earlier times. What the great men of the Classical period did was to lay the foundations of surgery as a science as well as an art. Surgery began to be based on the bedrock of anatomy and physiology and on a closer study of the reactions of the human body to disease and injury. The supreme importance of diagnosis was recognized: methods of physical examination became more thorough, careful case histories began to be kept, a literature of surgery came into being, and it was possible to compare personal experience with that of others. The technique of performing some operations was greatly improved, but there are few references to measures for the alleviation of pain.

FOR FURTHER READING

Allbutt, Sir C. *Greek Medicine in Rome.* 1921.

Caton, R. *The Temples and Ritual of Asklepios.* 1900.

Celsus. *De Medicina. With an English Translation by W. G. Spencer.* (Loeb Classical Library). 3 vols. 1935–8.

Gordon, B. L. *Medicine throughout Antiquity.* Philadelphia. 1949.

Hamilton, A. *Incubation, or the Cure of Disease in Pagan Temples and Christian Churches.* St. Andrews. 1906.

Hippocrates. *Works, with an English Translation by W. H. S. Jones and E. T. Withington.* (Loeb Classical Library). 4 vols. 1923–31.

Milne, J. S. *Surgical Instruments in Greek and Roman Times.* 1907.

Neuburger, M. *History of Medicine.* Vol. 1. 1910.

Singer, C. *Greek Biology and Greek Medicine.* 1922.

Withington, E. T. *Medical History from the Earliest Times.* 1894.

Wood, S. Homer's surgeons: Machaon and Podalirius. *Lancet,* 1931, i, 992, 947.

CHAPTER FOUR

The Middle Ages

FOR a thousand years following the collapse of the Roman Empire little progress was made in either the art or the science of medicine. There were no medical schools in Western Europe and very few physicians. Those who had studied medicine at all seriously were members of the Church. Unfortunately blind adherence to authority as fostered by the early Christian Church tended to inhibit freedom of thought and observation. Furthermore, because the human body was held sacred, dissection was prohibited and this meant that the sciences of anatomy and physiology, which are the bedrock of all medical knowledge, could not be studied in a practical manner.

A close connexion between religion and medicine had existed, as we have already seen, among primitive peoples and in the earliest civilizations. With the spread of Christianity medicine again became the concern of the priestly caste. One of the first principles of Christianity was the healing of the sick, but disease was regarded in the main as something to be endured with patience and resignation. Investigation into the natural causes of disease was discouraged. Such treatment as there was consisted of quiet and rest in a peaceful atmosphere, intercession, prayer and the cult of healing saints. Churches and shrines dedicated to certain saints and martyrs became places of pilgrimage. The number of saints associated with the healing art is legion. A patron saint was usually regarded as having power to relieve affections of a particular organ or part of the body.

Thus Saint Apollonia was the patron saint of those suffering from toothache because when she was martyred all her teeth were pulled out by huge pincers; Saint Agatha was concerned with diseases of the breast because her breasts were cut off; Saint Sebastian and Saint Roch were plague saints; Saint Blaze, Bishop of Sebaste in Armenia (c. A.D. 316) was invoked in all diseases of the throat because he had cured a boy who had swallowed a fish bone. On this saint's day—3 February—the ceremony of the Benediction of the Throat is still carried out at St. Ethelreda's Church in the City of London.

The most famous of all medical saints are Cosmas and Damian, Arabian twin brothers who were converted to Christianity. The brothers practised medicine and performed many marvellous cures before being martyred in A.D. 303 because they would not forswear their faith. They became the patron saints of barbers, surgeons and apothecaries and representations of them are found in the coats of arms of many medical bodies at the present day. The most celebrated miracle of healing performed by Cosmas and Damian was the amputation of a cancerous leg and its replacement by the leg of a Moor who had just died. This remarkable operation is shown in a very beautiful miniature painting which has been ascribed to the famous artists Andrea and Francesco Mantegna.

The practice of surgery was forbidden to priests and it therefore passed almost entirely into the hands of barbers and other uneducated men, although there were always a few surgeons of higher rank who attended royalty and the nobility.

Such surgery as was attempted in the early part of the Middle Ages was meddlesome. There were itinerant operators for stone, cataract and hernia, but surgery consisted in the main in the treatment of wounds, fractures, and dislocations. Other operations are described in surgical texts but it is doubtful if they were ever performed.

Curiously enough some of the surgical textbooks of the Middle Ages contain references to anaesthetic sponges which were prepared by soaking them in various herbs reputed to have soporific properties. The favourite herb for this purpose was the mandrake, the reputed effects of which were well known to Shakespeare who makes Cleopatra say:

"Give me to drink Mandragora
That I might sleep out this great gap of time
My Antony is away."

The Herbal of Dioscorides (first century A.D.) contains specific directions for giving a decoction of mandragora "to such as shall be cut or cauterized" and this is one of the earliest references to surgical anaesthesia. Bernard de Gordon (c. 1260–1308) tells us that the Salernitans rubbed up poppy seed and henbane and used them as a plaster to deaden the sensibility of a part to be cauterized. Arnold of Villanova (c. 1235–1311) has the following recipe: "To produce sleep so profound that the patient may be cut and will feel nothing, as though he were dead, take of opium, mandragora bark, and henbane root equal parts, pound them together and mix with water. When you want to sew or cut a man dip a rag in this and put it to his forehead and nostrils. He will soon sleep so deeply that you may do what you will. To wake him up, dip the rag in strong vinegar." Hugh of Lucca's method was an improved version of this. He added the juice of lettuce, ivy, mulberry, sorrel, and hemlock to the above and boiled the whole with a new sponge. This was then dried and when wanted dipped in hot water and applied to the patient's nostrils. But if the medieval surgeons made use of anaesthetics it seems that their knowledge died with them. After the medieval period there is no evidence whatever for the use of anaesthetic drugs until the nineteenth century.

The progress of surgery was long retarded by the belief that suppuration was an essential process in the healing of wounds. Wounds were treated with all kinds of messy and obnoxious ointments and preparations and were kept open by artificial means. The use of the ligature to control haemorrhage had been well known to the Greeks, but it was abandoned by many later surgeons in favour of cauterization with red hot irons or the application of boiling oil. The miracle is that any patients survived these horrors, but operations were never performed except in cases of extreme need and when the patient's sufferings made any attempt at relief welcome. Not all surgeons favoured meddlesome and brutal methods; a few enlightened men advocated simple dry dressings and other conservative measures. Lack of exact anatomical and physiological knowledge was a tremendous handicap, but the extensive experience gained in the wars of the period gave many surgeons a high degree of skill in the management of wounds and injuries of the simpler type.

The first medical school in the west arose at Salerno, the beautiful seaside town some thirty-five miles south of Naples, which was the scene of such bitter fighting in the late war. According to legend the Salerno school was founded by four Masters—a Jew, a Greek, an Arab and a Latin. It seems that the school came into being in the ninth century and that it reached its zenith in the eleventh. There was a regular curriculum of study extending over five years, after which the candidate had to undergo an examination. Successful students were then entitled to call themselves Doctor and to practise. A very interesting fact is that there were apparently several women doctors who taught at Salerno. The eleventh and twelfth centuries saw the rise of the great universities of Western Europe, the earliest of which were those of Paris, Bologna, Oxford, Montpellier, Cambridge and Padua. Medical schools came into existence in all these universities but medicine was not really regarded as a subject worthy of study for its own sake. For a long time it was taught as a branch of philosophy and was part of the knowledge that any learned man was expected to acquire. Medical teaching was almost entirely bookish, consisting in the reading and expounding of the ancient Greek authorities. Ideas as to the causation of disease were bound up with the theories of the "elements" and the "humours" and with astrology. The position of the stars governed diagnosis, prognosis and treatment, and caused particular maladies. There were propitious and non-propitious times for blood letting, for the administration of medicines, and for attempting surgical operations. Before condemning the medieval doctor we should remember that similar superstitious ideas regarding health and disease are rampant today, and there never was a time when people "poured so many substances of which they know little into bodies of which they know less".

All that has been said above in regard to medical education applied to physicians. Physicians were all learned men, graduates in art and in medicine; they never carried out any manual procedure. With a few exceptions, surgeons were an inferior body of craftsmen whose education and training was undertaken by their own guilds. The university of Bologna was one of the few centres at which surgical teaching was carried on at a higher level. Here worked Hugh of Lucca and his son Theodoric of Cervia. Hugh served with the Bolognese in Syria and Egypt during the Crusades. He died in 1252 leaving a great reputation. None of his writings have survived but they are quoted by his son. Theodoric, like many of the leading medical men of his time, was a member of the Church; he belonged to the Dominican Order and was at one time Bishop of Cervia. He wrote a "Chyrurgia" of marked originality. He was the first to use simple dressings for the treatment of wounds, maintaining that the formation of pus was not necessary and that complicated and messy applications hindered healing. Theodoric also describes the use of the soporific sponge to produce sleep during surgical operations. It may be claimed that Theodoric was a pioneer of both antisepsis and anaesthesia and the originator of ideas which did not meet with general acceptance until six centuries later. In accordance with the custom of the age Theodoric includes a number of religious formulae in his surgery: "To extract arrows from the body repeat three Paternosters, then take the arrows between the joined hands and say 'Nicodemus, drew out the nails from the hands and feet of the Lord', and it will at once come out." The Bishop admits that he has never tried this himself but he has been assured of its efficacy by many reliable persons.

Another great teacher of Bologna was William of Saliceto (1210–77). He was one of those who aimed at the reunion of medicine and surgery. He sutured nerves that had been severed and differentiated the spurting arterial blood from venous haemorrhage. Unlike the Arab surgeons he preferred the knife to the cautery. He describes a case which he saw when serving as a young army surgeon: "I saw a soldier of Bergamo struck by a great arrow from a machine. The arrow went in on the right side of the neck near the vessels, but without injuring them, and came out over his left shoulder. I extracted it in the way described in the chapter on Arrow Wounds of the Head and treated the wound in the manner often related. The man got perfectly well and lived long after and I got a good fee." Like many of the early surgical writers William of Saliceto offers his readers some advice on the conduct of their practice. Surgeons, he said, should be "reflective, quiet, and with downcast countenance, giving an impression of wisdom. They should have little conversation with the patient's friends and relatives."

Lanfranc of Milan (d. 1315) became the head of the French school of surgery. He was associated with a corporation of surgeons called the Collège de St. Côme which he had organized some time before 1260. In the year 1296 he finished a large treatise on surgery which was not however printed until 1490. Lanfranc was a careful observer and a skilful operator. Unlike William of Saliceto he preferred the cautery to the knife but he advised caution in the performance of such operations as trephination, the removal of cataract, lithotomy, and hernia. He deplored the fact that blood letting and other minor operations were often left to the barbers and maintained that "No one can be a good physician if he is ignorant of surgical operations, and no one can perform operations if he does not know medicine." It is recorded of him that when a child fell with a knife in his hand and wounded a vein in the neck, Lanfranc held his finger to the spot for an hour while an assistant fetched a styptic of frankincense, aloes, white of egg, and hare's fur.

Lanfranc quotes the view of Hippocrates that wounds of the brain, heart, lung, bladder, stomach, and small intestines are fatal. If therefore a surgeon is called to such a case shall he run away? He replies that if in his own country and of established reputation the surgeon should do his best for his patient after giving due warning to the friends, otherwise he should by all means avoid such cases. The lack of surgical enterprise shown at this period is understandable enough in view of the decided risk for the surgeon if his patient was so ungracious as to die under his hands. Many practitioners refused to undertake dangerous cases unless indemnified against failure. About A.D. 1250 a nobleman of Bologna was injured in the side so severely that a portion of his lung protruded through the wound. For some time no one could be found to undertake the case, till at last an appeal was made to the two most famous operators of the age, Hugh of Lucca and Roland of Parma. Those intrepid surgeons, having obtained permission of the Bishop and taken an oath from thirty of the patient's friends that no harm would happen to them, boldly excised the protruding lung and applied a consolidative powder. The patient recovered and went on a pilgrimage to Jerusalem.

In many early legal codes a medical man was required to enter into a contract and give pledges before undertaking a case. The Visigothic code contains the enactment: "If a physician injures a freeman by bleeding, let him pay 10 solidi; but if the patient dies, let him be handed over to his relatives to treat as they please. If a slave is injured or killed the physician shall replace him by one of equal value." This and similar drastic laws remind us of the code of Hammurabi of two thousand years earlier. These were not empty threats. There are many records of physicians and surgeons being executed because they failed to cure illustrious patients. Jean d'Amand, a barber-surgeon, who was accused of trying to poison Pope John XXII, was flayed alive. In 1337, just before the blind King John of Bohemia went to fight and fall at Crécy, a travelling oculist offered to cure him of his blindness. He failed and was promptly sewn up in a sack and thrown into the River Oder. In 1464 King Matthias of Hungary was wounded by an arrow the head of which remained in his arm. He made a proclamation like those in fairy tales, that whoever cured him should have great reward but he who failed should lose his life. For four years no one ventured, then came Hans of Dokenburg in Alsace and got out the iron. The king gave him great gifts and made him a knight, but we are not told whether he married the king's daughter!

A famous pupil of William of Saliceto was Henri de Mondeville (1260–1320). He was surgeon to Philip the Fair and Louis X of France and taught at Montpellier. He stressed the knowledge of anatomy and his surgical practice was in advance of his times. He used ligation instead of the cautery and was one of those who taught that suppuration was a hindrance to wound healing. He advised the dry treatment of wounds, but hesitated to adopt new operations because "it is dangerous for a surgeon, who is not of repute, to operate in any way different to that method in common use". De Mondeville did not always follow the highest standards of professional conduct.

In order to sustain the spirits of a patient he suggested that "false letters may be written telling of the death of his enemies, or if he is a Canon of the Church, he is elected". Another more reputable means of cheering up a despondent patient was to "solace him by playing on a ten string psaltery". He expected to be well paid for his services. "When treating an accident, the friends should be excluded as they may faint and cause a disturbance; nevertheless, sometimes a higher fee may be obtained from persons fainting and breaking their heads than from the principal patient." He seems to have had a keen sense of humour and suggests that if a physician were attending a long and difficult case without result he should say, "My business prevents me from attending you any longer, so I advise you to call in a surgeon."

Anatomical dissection began to be practised towards the end of the thirteenth century, first at Bologna about 1281 and then at Padua, Venice, Florence, Montpellier and other centres. The first practical manual of anatomy was written in 1316 by Mondino de Luzzi who taught at Bologna. The dissections were chiefly the bodies of executed criminals, but they were sometimes more in the nature of autopsies done to establish the cause of death especially in cases of suspected poisoning. The actual dissection was carried out by a surgeon or barber-surgeon under the superintendence of a physician. The practice of dissection had become sufficiently important at Padua to justify the building of a special anatomical theatre about 1446.

The only case of human vivisection for which there seems fairly good evidence dates from a later period, and is related in John of Troyes' *History of Louis XI*:

"In January, 1474, an archer of Meudon was condemned for many robberies, and especially for robbing the church at Meudon, to be hanged at Paris. He appealed to the Parlement which confirmed the sentence. Then the physicians and surgeons of the city represented to the king that many and divers persons were grievously molested and tormented by stone, colic, and pains in the side, with which the said archer was also much troubled, and that Mon-

seigneur du Bouchaige (a favourite courtier mentioned by
Comines) was sorely afflicted by the said maladies, and that
it would be very useful to see the places where these maladies
are concreted, and that this could be best done by vivi-
secting a human being, which could be well effected on the
person of the said archer, who was also about to suffer death.
Which opening and incision was accordingly done on the
body of the said archer, and the place of the said maladies
having been sought out and examined, his bowels were
replaced and he was sewn up again. And by the king's
command the wound was well dressed, so that he was
perfectly healed within a fortnight, and he received a free
pardon, and some money was given him as well."

The most famous surgeon of the later Middle Ages was
Guy de Chauliac (1300–67). He studied at Montpellier and
Bologna, but most of his life was spent at Avignon where he
was physician and chaplain to Pope Clement VI and two of
his successors. He was a learned man and his writings were
based upon observation and experience. His *Chirurgia Magna*
was written in Latin and then printed in French in 1478. In
one respect he was rather retrograde in that he advocated the
use of salves and plasters and of the cautery in place of simple
dressings. In other respects he was a reformer and he had high
ethical principles. "A good surgeon should be courteous,
sober, pious, and merciful, not greedy of gain, and with a
sense of his own dignity." He was interested in the radical
cure of hernia but did not advise operation in every case, pre-
ferring the use of a truss whenever possible. In speaking of
fractures of the thigh he writes: "After the application of
splints, I attach to the foot a mass of lead as a weight, taking
care to pass the cord which supports the weight over a small
pulley in such a manner that it shall pull on the leg in a
horizontal direction." He also suspended a rope above the bed
of the patient so as to facilitate change of position. He may have
been the first to employ extension in the treatment of fractures.
He insisted on the importance of anatomy "without which one
can do nothing in surgery". He was opposed to leaving the
surgery of hernia, stone, and cataract to itinerant quacks. In

penetrating wounds of the abdomen he advises that any impaired internal organ should be drawn out (enlarging the external wound if necessary), cleansed, sutured, and gently replaced. He refers to the method of suturing by means of ants' heads, but condemns it. He himself recommends the use of "furrier's stitches". Guy de Chauliac made noteworthy contributions to dentistry, giving rules for the care and cleansing of the teeth so as to prevent decay and advising replacement of lost teeth by other human teeth or by artificial dentures made of bone.

Guy's book contains an historical sketch of surgery. He describes various instruments and the proper contents of a surgical case. This should contain six instruments: scissors, speculum, razor, scalpel, needle, and lancet. Guy describes five methods of controlling haemorrhage: suture, tamponade, compression, ligature and cautery. He recognized nature as the chief workman whom the surgeon assists by removing foreign bodies, bringing together separated parts and in other ways.

In most other countries of Europe surgery was still in a primitive state. Only one British surgeon of note belongs to this period, John of Arderne (1307–90) who studied at Montpellier, practised in France for some years, and was present at the battle of Crécy. On his return to England he practised first at Newark and then in London. He was a specialist in the treatment of rectal disorders and practised an operation for the cure of fistula. This consisted in boldly incising the wall of the fistula and checking bleeding by the pressure of sponges. He recognized cancer of the rectum and noted that treatment could only be palliative. His practice was mainly amongst the wealthy nobles and true merchant class. He travelled long distances to operate and charged high fees. He declares that he never took less than 100 shillings (£68 13s. 4d.) for the cure of an anal fistula together with an annual pension of 100 shillings—immense fees considering the value of money at that time. But as all the world does not suffer from anal fistula the surgeon must be prepared to earn his living by carrying out minor operations. Arderne declares that everybody would be immensely benefited by taking an enema twice or thrice yearly. The operation should be performed by a master such as himself, with his new and improved syringes, and he concludes with a list of fees. Although Arderne evidently had an eye to the main chance, he set a high moral standard, advising surgeons to cultivate modesty, charity, and studious habits and to be scrupulously clean in dress and person. "When a sick man or any of his friends comes to the doctor to ask help or counsel of him he ought not to be either too rough or too familiar but pleasant in his bearing according to the position of the person, to some reverently, to some friendly, for the wise man says 'familiarity breeds contempt'. . . . A leech ought also to have well cut clothes, dressing soberly and not like a clown or a poet. He ought too to have clean hands and well shaped nails which should not be black or filthy. He should behave himself courteously at a lord's dining table and he should not offend the guests who are sitting near him either in words or in deeds. He should hear many things but speak little; the wise man says 'it is better to use the ears than the tongue.' "

John Arderne shared some of the superstitions of his time and he mentions various charms. Though he often quotes his predecessors he relies largely on his own experience of which the following is an example: "There was a man smitten on the shin, but the skin was not broken; but after the third day it swelled and began to grieve him; then he went unto one un-skilled, until he had in his leg a great round hole and deep [sic] and full of black filth like unto burnt flesh. So when he came to me I cured him thus. First I washed the place with white wine warmed, in which was sodden croppes of the herbe colewort, and juice of plantain. Afterwards I put to a plaster made of plantain, rhubarb, parsley, honey, rye meal and white of egg mingled together; the place being mundified I put to powder 'croeferoberon' with a plaster of black soap, sulphur and arsenic. If any man be smitten on any part of the leg violently without wounding, as often happens either by a horse or a stone or club or such like, it is good in the beginning to annoint the place and bring out the bruised blood thereof, and after to apply plasters repressing the pain and swelling. . . . Take for your cure as much as you can get, with good assurance for your money when you have done."

Arderne also records an interesting case of tetanus. "There

was a gardener who, while he worked amongst the vines, cut his hand with a hook upon a Friday after the feast of [the translation of] Saint Thomas of Canterbury in summer [7 July], so that the thumb was wholly separated from the hand except at the joint where it was joined to the hand, and it could be bent backward to his arm and there streamed out much blood.

"And as touching the cure. The thumb was first reduced to its proper position and sewn on and the bleeding was stopped with Lanfranc's red powder and the hairs of a hare and the dressing was not removed until the third day. When it was removed there was no bleeding. Then there was put upon it those medicines which engender blood, redressing the wound once every day. The wound began to purge itself and to pour out matter. And on the fourth night after, the blood began to break out about midnight and he lost almost two pounds of it by weight. And when the bleeding was stopped the wound was redressed daily as before. Also on the eleventh night about the same time the bleeding broke out again in greater quantity than it did the first time. Nevertheless the blood was staunched, and by the morning the patient was so taken with the cramp in the cheeks and in the arm that he was not able to take any meat into his mouth, nor could he open his mouth, and on the fifteenth day the bleeding broke out again, and on the eighteenth day the blood broke out again, beyond all measure, and always the cramp continued and he died on the twentieth day."

In the early Middle Ages the wounded soldier was looked after first by women camp followers or by those of his comrades who possessed some surgical skill and afterwards by professional surgeons. A number of physicians and surgeons were attached to the king's person while others formed part of the general levy; some young surgeons joined the army for the sake of the practice provided by a campaign and because of the booty which they could pick up. When Edward I invaded Scotland (1299–1301) he was accompanied by no less than seven medical men, including a king's physician with two juniors, a king's surgeon and two assistants, and a simple surgeon. The king's physician and surgeon were of high standing, receiving the pay of knights (two shillings a day). In the following century Nicholas Colnet, physician, and Thomas Morstede, surgeon, went with Henry V to Agincourt. Both were attended by three mounted archers and Morstede had twelve members of his own craft as his assistants. Colnet and Morstede were to receive one shilling and their attendants sixpence per day, together with a share of the plunder and their part of the usual bounty, viz. 100 marks per quarter for every thirty men during the actual campaign. If they got all this they were well paid indeed, but it is probable that their salaries were often in arrears. Another surgeon, William Bredwardyn, was afterwards associated with Morstede and they were allowed two wagons and a chariot for their baggage. Field hospitals and ambulances appear at the close of the Middle Ages. One of the best army medical services was the Spanish, introduced by Queen Isabella in the fifteenth century. She produced six large tents and their furniture, together with physicians, surgeons, medicines and attendants and commanded that they should charge nothing for she would pay for all.

At the end of the fifteenth century lived three German surgeons who had special experience of war surgery. Heinrich von Pfolspeundt was a Bavarian army surgeon who wrote a book on bandaging and the treatment of wounds in 1460. His main concern was with arrow wounds but it contains a first brief reference to the extraction of bullets and to plastic surgery of the face. A more detailed account of gunshot wounds was given by Jerome of Brunswick, in 1497. Hans von Gersdorff had forty years of experience of campaigns. His field book for the army surgeon appeared in 1517. He extracted bullets with special instruments and dressed the wound with warm, but not boiling oil. He enclosed amputation stumps in the bladder of an animal after checking the haemorrhage by pressure and styptics. The works of Brunswick and Gersdorff contains many striking illustrations of operation scenes, instruments and appliances. Artificial limbs were skilfully made at this period. Goetz von Berlichingen, a famous German knight, had his right hand shot away at the siege at Landshut in 1505. An iron one was substituted and he was known henceforth as Goetz of the Iron Hand.

As we have seen, many of the most distinguished surgeons of the Middle Ages were clerics, but the practice of medicine and surgery by members of the Church was not favoured by the hierarchy. Many laws were passed against the practice of medicine for worldly profit. In 1215 the Fourth Lateran Council forbade all sub-deacons, deacons or priests to practise that part of surgery that had to do with burning and cutting, and finally Pope Honorius III prohibited all persons in holy orders from practising medicine in any form. These decrees had little effect and many distinguished clerical surgeons carried on with their work.

The final separation of medicine from the Church was probably due to more general causes, such as the increasing complexity of the art, the rise of the great secular universities, and the fact that many of the recognized medical textbooks were translations from the works of disbelieving Moslems.

During the Dark Ages that followed the final collapse of the Roman Empire medicine was at a very low ebb in Western Europe. Both medicine and surgery were, however, extensively cultivated in the great Arabic Empire founded by the prophet Mahomet. This empire lasted from the seventh to the thirteenth century and eventually stretched from Spain to Samarkand. Medicine had been studied at an even earlier period by the Arabs. Nestorius, patriarch of Jerusalem, was banished for heresy in A.D. 431 and, with a band of followers, fled to Edessa in Asia Minor where he went on to Jundi Shapur in Southwest Persia where there arose a very notable medical centre.

Although the names Arab and Arabian are generally applied to the language and to the physicians of the Moslem empire, very few were genuine Arabs. Some were Syrians and some Persians. Not all were even of the Moslem faith; many were Christians or Jews. In early times the Moslems were very tolerant towards other faiths and learning was greatly respected by them. At Jundi Shapur the Arabs learned much of Greek medicine and to it they added contributions of their own. They preserved many of the Greek medical texts by translating them into Persian and Arabic. In the early period of Arabian medicine Greek ideas were dominant. In the second period Arabian medicine reached its zenith and it produced some of the greatest figures in the history of medicine. The most renowned of all was Rhazes (865–925), a Persian, who was chief physician to the hospital at Baghdad. It is said that when he was asked to choose a site for this hospital, he hung pieces of meat at various points in the city, and selected the place at which putrefaction was longest delayed. One of his greatest achievements was to distinguish smallpox from measles. But he was also a pioneer in the use of animal gut for sutures and he introduced a number of new remedies such as mercurial ointment.

Isaac Judaeus, a contemporary of Rhazes, was an Egyptian Jew who practised in Tunisia. He wrote a "Guide for Physicians" which contains a number of pithy maxims such as: "Ask thy reward when the sickness is at its height, for being cured the patient will surely forget what thou didst for him," and "Treating the sick is like boring holes in pearls, and the physician must act with caution lest he destroy the pearl committed to his charge".

Arabian medicine reached its summit in Avicenna (A.D. 980–1037), who has been called the Prince of Physicians. He is said to have known the Koran by heart at the age of ten and to have been appointed Court Physician at eighteen. His tomb at Hamadan was restored recently and it is still a place of pilgrimage. Avicenna was one of the greatest sages of the East, but, like his contemporary Omar Kháyyam, he had a fondness for wine, women and song, and according to some biographers his life was shortened by alcoholic indulgence. However that may be, his reputation as a physician and philosopher was immense and his great textbook of medicine, known as the "Canon", was regarded as authoritative for hundreds of years.

The greatest surgeon of the Arabian school was Albucasis (died c. 1013). Albucasis was born near Cordova in Spain. His writings give an invaluable account of the surgery of the period and contain many pictures of instruments. Much of the work is based upon Paul of Aegina but it includes a great deal of personal observation.

Albucasis regrets that the Arabs had not made a proper study of anatomy and also that they had neglected Galen and the other classical writers. He himself constantly refers to Galen. The first part of his work has a great deal about the use of the cautery which he especially recommended in many surgical disorders. The second book treats of surgical operations and advises above all not to undertake any operation without knowing the cause of the malady and without having worked out all the steps of the operation in advance. He recommends the surgeon never to forget that God is watching his work and that he therefore should never operate merely for the sake of gain.

He gives interesting indications for lithotomy, herniotomy, and for the treatment of abdominal wounds. For injuries of the intestine he recommends holding together the edges of the wound and suturing by means of large ants. He gives detailed descriptions of trephining, amputations, operations for fistula, goitre, and aneurysm. He has interesting sections on dentistry, and recommends the use of artificial teeth made of bone. For disorders of the bladder he recommends the use of a silver catheter instead of the bronze catheter that had been used up to that time. Various sutures for wounds are described, including the double suture, and instruments are specified in detail. Fractures and dislocations are well treated but in this section he leans heavily upon Galen. One of his sayings was, "Surgical operations are of two kinds, those that benefit the patient and those which usually kill him." That he was a conservative surgeon is evident from the motto "Caution" with which he begins and ends his book.

Albucasis seems to have given the first account of haemophilia. "I have found men in a certain village who told me that whenever they suffered a severe wound, it bled till they were dead, and they added that when a child rubbed his gums they began to bleed, and went on bleeding till he died. Another also having had a vein opened by a phlebotomist bled to death; and they said that, in general, most of them died thus. I have never seen such a thing save in this village; nor do I find it noticed in ancient writers. I know not the cause of it, but as for the cure, I suppose a cautery should be applied at once; but I have never tried it and the whole thing is marvellous to me."

The teaching and practice of medicines were highly organized under the Moslems. There was a large hospital at Baghdad in the time of the Caliph Harun-Al-Raschid (of Arabian Nights fame). At the height of the empire there were large hospitals in all the great centres. In the Cairo hospital, founded in 1283, there were special divisions for the wounded, for eye patients, for those with fever (in whose rooms the air was refreshed with fountains), and for gynaecological cases. It also included a large library, an orphanage, and a chapel where fifty chaplains recited the Koran day and night without intermission for all who chose to hear. Musicians and story-tellers were provided for the benefit of those troubled with sleeplessness, and the convalescent received at his departure five pieces of gold that he might not be obliged to return to work immediately. The hospital was directed by a chief physician, who had other subordinant physicians under him and there were male and female nurses. Daily lessons were given to the students and they had to pass strict examinations.

It cannot be said that the Arabs made outstanding contributions to surgery. They were very fond of cauterizing with red hot irons. Eye diseases, very prevalent in the East, also claimed much of their attention, but their greatest achievements were in medical treatment. They excelled in chemistry and were the inventors of many processes—such as distillation and sublimation—connected with the preparation of drugs. Among the common drugs which they introduced were benzoin, camphor, senna, musk and laudanum.

FOR FURTHER READING

Browne, E. G. *Arabian Medicine.* 1921.

Elgood, C. *A Medical History of Persia.* Cambridge, 1951.

Ellis, E. S. *Ancient Anodynes.* 1946.

Fletcher, R. Diseases bearing the names of Saints. *Bristol med.-chir. J.,* 1912, *30,* 289.

Fülöp-Miller, R. *Triumph over Pain.* 1938.

Gask, G. *Essays in the History of Medicine.* 1950.

Gruner, O. C. *The Canon of Medicine of Avicenna.* 1921.

Lanfranc. *Science of Cirurgie.* (Early English Text Society). 1894.

Mercier, C. A. *Astrology and Medicine.* 1914.

Packard, F. R. *The School of Salerno.* Oxford. 1922.

Power, Sir D. *De Arte Phisicali et de Cirurgia of Master John Arderne.* 1922.

Riesman, D. *Story of Medicine in the Middle Ages.* 1935.

Singer, C. *From Magic to Science*. 1928.

Singer, C. and D. On a miniature ascribed to Mantegna of an operation by Cosmas and Damian. *Contributions to Medical and Biological Research presented to Sir William Osler*. New York, 1919, Vol. 1, p. 166.

Theodoric. *The Surgery of Theodoric. Translated by E. Campbell and J. Colton*. New York. 1955.

Walsh, J. J. *Mediaeval Medicine*. 1900.

CHAPTER FIVE

The Renaissance

THAT great turning point in the history of civilization known as the Renaissance was accompanied by profound changes in medicine and surgery as in all other departments of knowledge. One of the most striking results of the new-found freedom of thought was an interest in the structure and function of the human body. In surgical practice lack of anatomical knowledge had been a great obstacle. Most early peoples, including the Greeks, had an instinctive fear of the dead and they attached great importance to the proper burial of bodies. Although they had obtained some little knowledge of bones and joints in connexion with the investigation of fractures and dislocations, the internal organs were to them a closed book.

Dissection of the human body was first practised systematically at the great medical school of Alexandria, which flourished from about 300 B.C. until the death of its last ruler, Cleopatra, in 30 B.C. After the decline of Alexandria dissection was carried on at a few other centres in the Middle East, but in the first two centuries of the Christian era human bodies were replaced by those of apes and other animals. The anatomical knowledge gained from the dissection of animals was probably a fairly adequate guide to such operative procedures as were carried out at this period because the abdomen, chest and the head were rarely opened by the surgeon's knife.

Anatomical demonstrations of a kind were introduced into some Italian medical schools early in the fourteenth century but their main purpose was to serve as an aid in memorizing what Galen had written a thousand years earlier. At this time, and for long after, the procedure was for the professor to read from some second- or third-hand manuscript version of Galen while a demonstrator pointed to the part under discussion with a wand. The actual dissection, which was carried out cursorily —for good and obvious reasons—was performed by a lowly

barber-surgeon. As the text of Galen was often based on the
dissection of an ape or a pig, there were naturally many
occasions when the anatomical structure under examination
did not correspond with Galen's description. But this did not
lead to the rejection of the ancient author because the teacher
explained that the human body had changed since Galen's
time!

Among the first to take up the scientific study of anatomy
were some of the great artists—Donatello, Michelangelo,
Raphael and that universal genius Leonardo da Vinci. All of
these engaged in dissection, using the scalpel before taking up
the brush or the pencil. Leonardo set out to study the bones
and muscles in relation to art but his interest grew and he
made important contributions to the anatomy and physiology
of the brain and of the internal organs, especially of the heart
and blood vessels. More than 750 of Leonardo's anatomical
sketches in red chalk are preserved in the Royal Library at
Windsor and they are perhaps the first accurate delineations
of the human body. Only the fact that the Leonardo drawings
were not reproduced in book form until recent times prevents
the great artist from being regarded as the true founder of
modern anatomy. This distinction belongs to Andreas Vesalius
(1514–64), a native of Brussels who studied medicine in Paris
and later taught surgery and anatomy at Padua and Bologna.

Vesalius was filled with a passionate desire for anatomical
study—even as a boy he had dissected mice and other small
animals—and many stories are told of the great risks which he
took in obtaining material. The supply of subjects for dissection
was still hopelessly inadequate and there is little doubt that
Vesalius was often forced to resort to unorthodox and highly
dangerous methods. On one occasion he stole the skeleton of a
criminal which was hanging on a gallows outside the city wall
of Louvain and the trophy proved of great value in his studies.
In 1543 when he was only twenty-eight years of age Vesalius
published his great work, *On the Fabric of the Human Body*. In
this magnificent folio volume the detailed descriptions of Vesalius are matched by the wonderfully exact and spirited woodcut illustrations which were drawn by Stephen van Calcar,
a pupil of Titian. For the first time in the history of medicine

doctors had at their disposal a detailed and accurate anatomical text with illustrations from the hand of a great artist. It was not to be expected that Vesalius would produce a work that was entirely free from errors, but his book is the foundation stone of anatomy—indeed of all modern medicine—because without a sound knowledge of the structure of the body there could be no real understanding of its functions in health and disease.

Vesalius was a practising surgeon as well as an anatomist. In July 1559 he was called into consultation when Henry II of France was wounded in a joust with the Count of Montgomery. The Count's lance had entered the King's visor and pierced the forehead. The court physicians and surgeons extracted several large splinters of wood and dressed the wound, but couriers were sent far and wide to summon further expert medical aid. Vesalius hurried from Brussels to Paris and was placed in charge of the case. In order to find out the possible extent of the injury experimental thrusts were made with lances on the heads of four criminals who had been decapitated on the previous day. In spite of all that could be done the King died on the eleventh day after the injury. Vesalius carried out a very thorough post-mortem examination which showed that the brain had suffered considerable damage and that a fatal outcome was inevitable.

The surgeons of the Renaissance gained wide experience in the religious wars of the period. They had many new problems to face, including that of the treatment of wounds caused by firearms. The French used gunpowder at the siege of Puiguillaume in 1338 but cannon were used by the English at the Battle of Crécy in 1346. Gunshot wounds did not become at all common however till some time after the introduction of the arquebus in the fifteenth century. The first surgeons to refer to such wounds are Pfolspeundt in 1460, Jerome of Brunswick, whose book of surgery was printed in 1497, and Hans von Gersdorff in 1517. Gunshot wounds at that time were caused by large missiles of low velocity. They caused ragged wounds and carried pieces of clothing into the tissues. These wounds were severe and were very liable to become septic. The universal belief among surgeons of the period was that gunpowder itself was venomous. To neutralize its effect the general practice was to cauterize the wound by injecting boiling oil. Jerome of Brunswick's book contains pictures of instruments for dilating and enlarging wounds in order to facilitate the injection of oil and the exit of discharges. Bleeding also was still controlled by the use of hot irons or boiling oil and wounds were daubed with all kinds of noxious and messy dressings which encouraged sepsis.

The first man to break away from the old doctrine that "diseases not curable by iron are curable by fire" was Ambroise Paré (1510–90), one-time barber's apprentice and later a dresser at the great Paris hospital, the Hôtel Dieu. Paré became the greatest military surgeon of all time. He began his service career in 1536 and followed the French armies in France, Flanders, Italy and Germany during the greater part of the next forty years. In his very first campaign he made a discovery which revolutionized the treatment of wounds at that time. This is Paré's graphic description of what happened after the French troops had captured the castle of Villaine:

"At that time I was a fresh water soldier, I had not yet seen wounds made by gunshot at the first dressing. It is true, I had read in 'John de Vigo', in the first book of wounds in general, the eighth chapter, that wounds made by weapons of fire did participate of venerosity, by reason of the powder, and for their cure command to cauterize them with oil of Elders scalding hot, in which should be mingled a little treacle; and not to fail, before I would apply of the said oil, knowing that such a thing might bring to the patient great pain, I was willing to know first, before I applied it, how the other chirurgions did for the first dressing, which was to apply the said oil the hottest that was possible into the wounds, with tents and setons; insomuch that I took courage to do as they did. At last I wanted oil, and was constrained instead thereof to apply a digestive of yolk of eggs, oil of roses, and turpentine. In the night I could not sleep in quiet, fearing some default in not cauterizing, that I should find those to whom I had not used the burning oil dead impoisoned; which made me rise very early to visit them, where beyond my expectation I found those to whom I had applied my digestive medicine, to feel little pain, and their wounds without inflammation or tumour, having rested reasonable well in the night: the other to whom was used the said burning oil, I found them feverish with great pain and tumour about the edges of their wounds. And then I resolved with myself never so cruelly to burn poor men wounded with gunshot."

Paré was still not happy about his treatment of gunshot wounds and he took every opportunity of picking up hints from older and more experienced men. "Being at Turin," he tells us, "I found a chirurgion, who had the fame above all others, for the curing of wounds of gunshot, into whose favour I found means to insinuate myself, to have the receipt of his balm, as he called it wherewith he dressed wounds of that kind, and he held me off the space of two years, before I could possibly draw the receipt from him. In the end by gifts and presents he gave it me, which was this, to boil young whelps new pupped, in oil of lilies, prepared earth worms, with turpentine of Venice. Then was I joyful and my heart made glad, that I had understood his remedy, which was like to that which I had obtained by great chance. See then how I have learned to dress wounds made with gunshot, not by books."

In 1552, Paré, now a surgeon of great experience, was serving in Germany. The following case illustrates both his skill and his humanity:

"One of the servants of a captain of the company of Monsieur de Rohan went with others thinking to enter into a church where the peasants were retired, thinking to find victuals by force or love: but amongst the rest was well beaten, and returned with seven wounds with a sword in the head; the least of which penetrated the second table of the skull, and he had four other upon the arms, and upon the right shoulder, which cut more than one half of the blade-bone or omoplate. He was brought back to his master's lodging, to seeing of him so wounded, and that they were to depart thence the morrow after at the break of day, and not thinking ever he could be cured, made him a grave, and would have cast him therein, saying that or else the peasants would massacre and kill him. I, moved with pity, told him that he might yet be cured if he were well dressed: divers gentlemen of the company prayed him that he would cause him to be brought along with the baggage, seeing I had the willingness to dress him; to which he agreed, and after that I had clothed him, he was put into a cart upon a bed well covered and well accommodated, which one horse did draw. I did the office of a physician, apothecary, chirurgion, and cook; I dressed him even to the end of his cure, and God cured him, in so much that all these three companies admired at this cure. The horsemen of the company of Monsieur de Rohan, the first muster that was made, gave me each one Crown, and the archers half a Crown."

The following story relating to an incident which occurred at the siege of Metz in 1552 illustrates both the new type of injury caused by gunshot and the credulity of the time:

Monsieur de La Roch-upon-Yon, one of the nobles serving in the Emperor's army, befriended Paré, who had been smuggled into the city with a message from the French king. In the course of the siege one of this nobleman's staff had his leg broken by a cannon shot, and he was being treated by an impostor who said that he would cure the leg without touching it. La Roch asked Paré to see the wounded man. "I found him," says Paré, "in his bed, his leg bended and crooked, without any dressing upon it; because the gentleman promised him cure, having his name and his girdle, with certain words. The poor gentleman wept and cried with pain which he felt, nor sleeping either night or day, in four days: then I mocked at this imposture and false promise. Presently I did so nimbly restore and dress his leg, that he was without pain and slept all night, and since (thanks be to God) was cured, and is yet at this present living, doing service to the king. The said Lord of the Roch-upon-Yon sent me a tun of wine to my lodging, and bid tell me, when it was dronken he would send me another."*

In 1564 Paré was responsible for a second great reform when he reintroduced the ligation of blood vessels, a method which

---

* The method of treatment being followed by the impostor in this case is a good example of sympathetic magic. (See page 103).

had been used by the ancients but had fallen into abeyance. In amputating he now tied the great blood vessels instead of cauterizing them with hot irons. That the use of ligatures in amputation became standard practice with Paré is shown by the following story. We also see how surgeons provided practice for their apprentices.

"In the year 1583 the tenth day of December Toussant Posson born at Roinville, at this present dwelling at Beauvais near Dourdan, having his leg all ulcered, and all the bones ciriez'd and rotten, prayed me for the honour of God to cut off his leg by reason of the great pain which he could no longer endure. After his body was prepared I caused his leg to be cut off, four fingers below the rotula of the knee, by Daniel Poullet one of my servants, to teach him and to imbolden him in such works; and there he readily tied the vessels to stay the bleeding, without application of hot irons, in the presence of James Guillemeau, Ordinary Chirurgion to the King, and John Charbonell, master Barber Chirurgion of Paris: and during the cure was visited by Master Laffilé and Master Courtin, Doctors, Regents in the Faculty of Medicine at Paris. The said operation was made in the house of John Gohell, innkeeper, dwelling at the sign of the White Horse in the Greve. I will not here forget to say, that the lady princess of Montpensier, knowing that he was poor, and in my hands, gave him money to pay for his chamber and diet. He was well cured, God be praised, and is returned home to his house with a wooden leg."

This is how Paré treated a real emergency:

"A Sergeant of the Chastelet dwelling near S. Andrew des Arts, who had a stroke of a sword upon the throat in the Clarkes' meadow, which cut asunder the jugular vein externe. As soon as he was hurt he put his handkercher upon the wound, and came to look for me at my house, and when he tooke away his handkercher the blood leaped out with great impetuosity: I suddenly tied the vein toward the root; he by this means was stanched and cured thanks be to God."

Paré was prepared to take good advice from whatever source it came, as is shown by the following anecdote:

"One of the marshalls of Montejan, his kitchen boys, fell by chance into a cauldron of oil being even almost boiling hot. I being called to dress him went to the next apothecaries to fetch refrigerating medicines commonly used in this case. There was present by chance a certain old countrywoman, who hearing that I desired medicines for a burn, persuaded me at the first dressing that I should lay to raw onions beated with a little salt; for so I should hinder the breaking out of blisters or pustules, as she had found by certain and frequent experience. Wherefore I thought good to try the force of her medicine upon this greasy skuleon. I the next day found those places of his body whereto the onions lay, to be free from blisters, but the other parts which they had not touched to be all blistered."

It is interesting to find that Paré refers to an operation for the correction of gross enlargement of the breasts. According to his predecessors, Paul of Aegina and Albucasis, it was possible to make a cross incision, remove the superfluous fat, and close the wound by stitching. Paré's caustic comment is that this is "to flay a woman alive, which I have never practised, nor counsel it to be done by the young surgeon." The great surgeon's conservative attitude is understandable, but operations of this kind are sometimes necessary and under present-day conditions they are frequently performed with complete success.

Paré was surgeon-in-ordinary to four kings of France. He was equally at home among the rigours of the camp or the luxurious atmosphere of the court. It was always Master Ambroise Paré who was sent for when a prince or nobleman was wounded but he gave equally diligent attention to the humblest soldier who needed his aid. At the time of the massacre of St. Bartholomew in 1572 Paré was the only Huguenot to be spared and that by direct order of the King. Paré exerted a great influence by his example and by his writings. His books were widely read because, unlike the majority of medical works of this period, they were in French and not in Latin; but he himself did not set too much store on book-learning. "Five things," he said, "are proper to the duty of a surgeon: to take away that which is superfluous; to restore to their places such things as are displaced; to separate those things which are joined together; to join those things which are separated; and to supply the defects of nature. Thou shalt far more easily and happily attain to the knowledge of these things by long use and much exercise, than by much reading of books or daily hearing of teachers. For speech how perspicuous and elegant soever it be, cannot so vividly express anything as that which is subjected to the faithful eyes and hands."

Paré was not only a very great surgeon but also a most attractive character. He possessed in fact all the attributes of the great surgeon—manual skill, experience, judgment, courage and compassion. His essential humility is shown in the famous saying (repeated many times in his books): "I dressed him and God healed him."

As we have seen one of the great merits of Ambroise Paré was that he set down his great experience and knowledge in the vulgar tongue. This example was followed in other countries, especially by the military surgeons. There was a great demand everywhere for concise practical manuals of war surgery on the part of the ordinary surgeons who were not highly educated men and could not read the great Latin tomes which form the textbooks of the time. Some of the early German surgeons who wrote practical books in their own language have already been mentioned. Another great name is that of Wilhelm Fabry of Hilden, a surgeon who gained much experience during the Thirty Years War. He is said to have introduced the tourniquet and to have amputated through healthy tissue in cases of gangrene.

During the Renaissance surgery began to attain a higher position than it had enjoyed in previous periods. Whereas it had been almost entirely in the hands of barbers it now began to be practised by men of a much higher standard of education and training. Among the most famous Italian surgeons of the period were Fabricius of Aquapendente, John of Vigo, and Guido Guidi of Pisa. Fabricius was professor of surgery at Padua and later also of anatomy. He ligated arteries and described techniques for tracheotomy, incision and drainage of the chest, and urethral surgery. His *Pentateuch of Surgery* (1592) contains illustrations of orthopaedic apparatus for the treatment of spinal curvature, wryneck, and so on. A prudent surgeon who avoided dangerous operations, he enjoyed great fame as a consultant and left a fortune of more than two hundred thousand ducats. John of Vigo was surgeon to Pope Julius II. His textbook of surgery, first published in 1514, passed through more than forty editions and was translated into French, Italian, Spanish, German and English. Believing that gunshot wounds were poisoned, he advised their treatment by cautery and by a plaster containing ground-up frogs, worms and vipers. The Surgery of Andrea della Croce (1573) contains some striking illustrations of operation scenes.

No account of Renaissance surgery would be complete without reference to the man who is regarded as the founder of modern plastic surgery. He was Gaspare Tagliacozzi of Bologna and his operation consisted in the transplantation of a flap of skin from the arm, the limb being bandaged in contact with the nose until the grafted part had established itself. This technique—which differed from the long forgotten Hindu method—was apparently evolved by the Brancas, a family of surgeons practising in Sicily in the first half of the fifteenth century. The Sicilian operation is thus referred to in a letter written to a friend in 1442 by the Italian poet Elisio Calenzio:

"Orpianus, if you wish to have your nose restored, come here. Really it is the most extraordinary thing in the world. Branca of Sicily, a man of wonderful talent, has found out how to give a person a new nose, which he either builds from the arm or borrows from a slave. When I saw this, I decided to write to you, thinking that no information could be more valuable. Now if you come, I would have you know that you shall return home with as much nose as you please. Fly!"

This letter, which was printed in 1503, helped to spread the belief that a nose could be transplanted from a slave or a voluntary "donor", but it is not possible to transfer skin or tissue from one human being to another—the grafts do not "take". It was, however, possible to make a nose or an ear by taking skin from the patient's own arm or forehead, and this operation Tagliacozzi practised with great success. In 1597 he published a beautifully illustrated book on rhinoplasty which ranks as the earliest treatise on plastic surgery. There was great need for these plastic operations in the sixteenth century owing to the frequent duels and street brawls; mutilation of the nose and ears was also a common form of punishment for theft, and it is probable that many noses were lost as a result of syphilis. After the time of Tagliacozzi the operation of rhinoplasty appears to have fallen into oblivion. It was not revived until the very end of the eighteenth century and then the impetus to its practice came not from the work of the famous surgery of Bologna but from that of the ancient Hindus.

The earliest known account of strangulated hernia was published by Pierre Franco, a celebrated Huguenot surgeon of Provence in 1556. Franco was at first one of the class of travelling cutters for the stone but he afterwards became a salaried surgeon of the republic of Berne. He bitterly laments the low estate of his fraternity. "The physicians and surgeons, even the apothecaries, can defend themselves when they are unfortunate, but if we have a mishap we must often run for our lives."

In no country was there a greater flowering of surgical talent than in England. Many examples of the surgical textbooks of the period have survived in the shape of books printed in "black letter" type and often illustrated with fascinating woodcut pictures. These books were written in the direct and picturesque language of the time. They were part of that great literature which is the principal glory of the Elizabethan age. From the scientific point of view they represent the first efforts to break away from the traditional teaching of the ancients and to present the results of original observation and experience.

Thomas Vicary (1495–1561) was the author of the first textbook of anatomy to be written in English. This bore the title, *A Treasure for Englishmen, containing the Anatomie of Man's Body* and was first published in 1548; it kept its place as a textbook until the seventeenth century. Vicary practised first at Maidstone as a barber-surgeon, and then in London, where he was soon recognized as one of the leading surgeons of the day.

He was appointed surgeon to Henry VIII and to St. Bartholomew's Hospital. In 1540 Vicary was instrumental in securing the king's assent to a union of the guilds of barbers and surgeons and he was elected the first Master of the new Barber-Surgeons' Company.

The barbers and surgeons of England had been organized in fraternities or guilds as early as the fourteenth century, the Barbers' Company of London being mentioned in records of 1308 and a Fellowship or Company of Surgeons having existed before 1369. The primary purpose of these associations was, like that of all trade guilds, to protect and promote the interests of their members. The guild supervised the recruitment, training and conduct of apprentices, laid down rules for the professional conduct of its members, and did all in its power to maintain a "closed shop". The fact that there were separate guilds of Barbers and Surgeons and that there was no overall supervision of the various forms of medical practice by the State led to endless trouble. The Barbers and the Surgeons quarrelled among themselves and they also came into collision with the Physicians and the Apothecaries. The Barbers had always practised minor surgery, such as blood-letting and tooth-drawing, and in time some of them began to take on more difficult work. This led to trouble with all the other associations and particularly with the Guild of Surgeons, whose members—men of much higher education and training—were doing all they could to raise the status of their profession. For a long time, however, the Barbers' Company was confirmed in its position and its privileges: the fact was that its members were acting as the general practitioners of the day and there was no other body of men to take their place. In 1540 a compromise was reached. By the Act of that year the two companies of Barbers and Surgeons were formally united under the name of the Masters or Governors of the Mystery and Commonalty of the Barbers and Surgeons of London, and it was declared that surgeons should no longer be barbers and that barbers should restrict their surgery to dentistry. The new company was empowered to impose fines upon unlicensed practitioners in London and was entitled to have the bodies of four executed criminals each year for the purpose of dissection. The united company—which is usually known by its short title of the Barber-Surgeons' Company—existed until 1745, when the union was dissolved, the Barbers and the Surgeons reverting to their former independent states. The Worshipful Company of Barbers still exists as one of the ancient Livery Companies of the City of London. The Company of Surgeons continued as the body responsible for the supervision of surgical practice but gradually lost its character as a City Company. In 1800 it was reconstituted by charter of George III as the Royal College of Surgeons of London and in 1843 Queen Victoria granted a new charter which changed its name to the Royal College of Surgeons of England.

The records of the old Barber-Surgeons' Company provide some interesting sidelights on the professional and social life of bygone London. One of the most important duties of the governing body of the Company was to straighten out difficulties between the master barber-surgeon and his apprentices. In some cases this meant the infliction of corporal punishment, as in the following from the Court Minutes of 22 August, 1569:

"Here was Richard Upton plaintif against his apprentice William Fish for that he ran away from his said Master the 20th of the former month and took with him certain instruments for surgery and other things more, which particulars were here presently seen and by the said Wm. Fish confessed, and that he had no cause to go from his said Master but that he would have gone to sea and according to his desert had correction and punishment unto ancient custom with rods."

On the other hand the Company watched over the interests of the apprentice and it would release him from his bond on production of sufficient evidence of neglect or ill-treatment. Thus on 30 June, 1601, Robert Wallis was "discharged from his apprenticeship for that it appeared to this Court that his Master did not maintain him with sufficient meat, drink and apparel."

On 15 October, 1573, the Court heard the complaint of John Staples who "brought his apprentice for evil behaviour by him committed in his Master's house with his Master's maid and he made his submission on his knees and asked his Master's forgiveness in the Court, and he was forgiven upon condition that he should amend well and faithfully without further complaint or else to have the punishment of the house."

On 27 April, 1556, it was ordered that no apprentice should wear a beard of beyond fifteen days' growth and that on breach of this order the Master of the apprentice was to pay a fine of half a mark. The worthy Barber-Surgeons seem to have taken a firm line in regard to the question of hair, as witness the treatment which they meted out to an apprentice who seems to have been the seventeenth-century equivalent of a Teddy boy:

"9 August 1647. Mr. Heydon complaining to this Court of his apprentice here present in Court for his evil and stubborn behaviour towards him and frequent absences out of his service in day time and in late hours at night. The said apprentice being in court to answer to the same did rudely and most irreverently behave himself towards his said Master and the whole Court in saucy language and behaviour using several oaths protesting that he will not serve his Master whatever shall come of it. The Court did therefore cause the hair of the said apprentice (being undecently long) to be cut shorter."

Apprenticeship lasted for at least seven years and provided an excellent course of practical training. At the expiration of his term the young surgeon had to attend at Barber-Surgeons' Hall for examination. There were three grades of licence: the first a limited licence to practise; the second a higher degree of Master of Anatomy and Surgery which carried a permanent licence to practise; and thirdly the Great Diploma, a qualification equivalent to the modern Fellowship of the Royal College of Surgeons. Surgical education did not end here for the members of the Barber-Surgeons' Company were obliged, under penalty of a fine, to attend the anatomical demonstrations and surgical lectures which were given in their Hall. By these means the practice and status of surgery were greatly advanced. A highly responsible body of trained surgeons arose—men who often quarrelled among themselves but who were dedicated to their profession and were united in their opposition to quackery.

John Banester (1533–1610) was one of the earliest teachers of anatomy to break away from the old traditions. He prac-tised with great reputation at Nottingham and later in London where he lectured at Barber-Surgeons' Hall in 1581. He was strongly in favour of the reunion of surgery with medicine, and wrote: "Some of late have fondly affirmed that the chirurgeon hath not to deal in physic. Small courtesy it is to break faithful friendship, for the one cannot work without the other, nor the other practise without the aid of both." This view of the essential unity of medicine was held by many of the newer school of surgeons, who saw the absurdity of treating a wounded limb as if it were something apart from the body of a man.

The Act of 1540 allowed the barber-surgeon to treat "all outward hurts and tokens of disease" but he was not permitted to administer medicine for "inward complaints". On the other hand, the physicians, who were a very small and exclusive body, did not compound drugs and never carried out manual procedures of any kind. If the patient needed to have an enema or if (as was almost certainly the case) he was to be "blooded", a barber-surgeon had to be fetched to do these simple things. Any medicines prescribed by the physician were supplied by a third party—the Apothecary, who in turn ob-tained his materials from a Druggist. This overlapping added enormously to the cost of sickness and was the cause of much jealousy between the different practitioners. In practice, of course, the strict letter of the law was rarely adhered to. The pure Physicians attended the Royal Family, the nobility, and the families of the wealthy city merchants; the higher grade of surgeons (who were also very few in number) drew the majority of their patients from the same classes of society; the ordinary Barber-Surgeons and, later, the Apothecaries attended to the ills of the common people and were in fact the general prac-titioners of the day.

Apart from those who had some legal right to practise medicine or surgery there were many who practised without any qualification or training whatsoever. In London and in the provinces there were swarms of quacks, empirics, mountebanks and itinerant operators for the stone, for hernia, and for cataract. The civic authorities often took stringent measures against these irregular practitioners, but so long as they did not stay too long in one place (and that was from all points of view inadvisable) they could continue their trade for years.

Thomas Gale (1507–87), a Tudor surgeon who saw much war service, describes the terrible conditions which he witnessed at Montreuil in 1544 under Henry VIII. He found sowgelders, tinkers and cobblers usurping the title and function of surgeons, and treating wounds with a horrible concoction used to grease the feet of horses and an ointment of shoemakers' wax and the rust of old kettles. Most of the wounded, even those with the most trivial injuries, perished. On returning from the wars Gale practised with great success in London and he became Serjeant-Surgeon to Queen Elizabeth. His writings, which are notable on account of their sound practical teaching, include *An Excellent Treatise on Wounds made with Gunneshot* (1563), and *Certaine Workes of Chirurgie, newlie compiled and published by Thomas Gale, Maister in Surgerie* (1586). Master Gale also left a striking picture of the maltreatment of the sick poor of this country by quacks and pretenders:

"In the year 1562 I did see in the two hospitals in London called St. Thomas' Hospital and St. Bartholomew's Hospital to the number three hundred and odd poor people that were diseased of sore legs, sore arms, feet and hands, with other parts of the body, so sore infected that a hundred and twenty of them could never be recovered without loss of a leg or of an arm, a foot or a hand, fingers or toes, or else their limbs crooked so that they were either maimed or else undone for ever. All these were brought to this mischief by witches, by women, by counterfeit javills [rascals] that take upon them to use the art, not only of robbing them of their money but of their limbs and perpetual health. And I, with certain other, diligently examining these poor people, how they came by their grievous hurts and who were their chirurgions that looked unto them and they confessed that they were either witches, which did promise by charms to make them whole, or else some women which would make them whole with herbs and suchlike things, or else some vagabond javill which runneth from one country to another promising unto them health only to deceive them of their money."

Another notable surgeon of Tudor England was William Clowes (1540–1604), surgeon to Queen Elizabeth and to St. Bartholomew's Hospital. He distinguished himself in service with the Army in Flanders and with the Navy against the Armada. His first book, published in 1579, was a treatise on venereal disease, the treatment of which formed an important part of the surgeon's practice at that time. The most important of his works is that on gunshot wounds; this first appeared in the year of the Great Armada and bore the lengthy title of *A Proved Practice for all young Chirurgians concerning Burnings with Gunpowder and Woundes made with Gunshot, Sword, Halbard, Pike, Launce, or such other.* Clowes was very much concerned with the question whether or not gunshot wounds were poisoned.

John Woodall (1569–1643) had extensive experience of surgery both afloat and ashore in the service of the East India Company and on the Continent. For some years he acted as surgeon to a colony of English merchants near Posen in Poland, and in 1604 he was sent as interpreter to the Tsar of Russia when James I was carrying on negotiations for the increase of our Muscovy trade. He wrote two very interesting books, *The Surgeon's Mate* (1617) and *Viaticum, or the Pathway to the Surgeon's Chest* (1628), which give valuable details of instruments and equipment and directions for their use. He invented a new kind of trephine for use in cranial surgery, but a greater claim to fame is his advocacy of lemon juice as a cure for scurvy—three hundred years before the discovery of vitamin C. As a surgeon, Woodall was strongly opposed to indiscriminate amputation. He believed that it was better to cut off a foot than a leg and even better to sacrifice a toe rather than a foot. Curiously enough, there is among the remarkable cases recorded by this conservative surgeon one of multiple amputation occurring in his practice at St. Bartholomew's Hospital:

"A history or a relation of a remarkable example of an amputation by me performed upon a woman in Saint Bartholomew's Hospital of both her legs, and part of seven of her fingers, in one morning together all taken off in the mortified part, without pain or loss of blood or spirits at all, and the woman was living at the writing hereof, and the patient was a certain poor maid or woman servant in London, named Ellen French, of whom there were made books and ballads, that were sung about the streets of her, namely, that whereas the said maid or servant was given to pilfering, and being accused thereof by her master and mistress, used to curse and swear and with words of execration to wish, that if she had committed the crime she stood accused of, that then her legs and hands might rot off, the which thing accordingly, no doubt by the providence of God, came to pass, as a judgement upon her, namely that both her legs almost to the gartering place, with parts of seven of her fingers did rot off, the which wretched woman nevertheless, being referred to me in Saint Bartholomew's Hospital to be cured, by God's mercy and permission, I healed her perfectly, but cutting off both her sphacelated legs in the mortified parts with also parts of her seven fingers, as is said, all in one morning without pain, terror or any loss of blood unto her, in the taking them off, and made her perfectly whole in a very short time, namely within three months, so merciful is God unto us vile creatures, when we are most unworthy of such his mercies."

Surgery in Scotland as elsewhere was in the hands of surgeons and barbers. In 1505 King James IV issued a decree setting up an Incorporation of Barber-Surgeons with certain rights and privileges. The guild was entitled to claim the body of one executed criminal each year for dissecting purposes, and it was to have the monopoly of making and selling *aqua vitae* (whisky) within the Burgh of Edinburgh. Both privileges have now lapsed! The Incorporation of Barber-Surgeons eventually became the Royal College of Surgeons of Edinburgh. James IV had a keen personal interest in medicine and surgery and was fond of exercising his amateur talents upon his subjects. His household accounts contain such items as: "To Dionynico, to gif the King leve to lat him bloud, 28s." and "To ane fallow because the King pullit furth his teth, 14s." In 1511 the King even operated upon one of his own barber-surgeons: "To Kynnard the barbour for twa teith drawn furth of his hed be the King, 14s." James limited himself to dressing wounds, blood-letting and the extraction of teeth—presumably he would have had to pay much higher fees to his patients if he had undertaken major surgery!

The most famous Scottish surgical author of the sixteenth century was Peter Lowe of Glasgow. His *Discourse on the Whole Art of Chirurgery* (1596) has some claim to be the first comprehensive textbook of surgery to be written in English. Lowe was a native of Glasgow who had spent more than twenty years in France and Flanders as a student and army surgeon and had then returned to practise in his native city. He was very anxious to unite all regular practitioners of medicine and surgery and to control the numerous quacks and charlatans. To this end he obtained from King James VI in 1599 a charter for the establishment of a Royal Faculty of Physicians and Surgeons of Glasgow. One of the original functions of this Faculty was the provision of free treatment for the poor. This trust, which appears to have been unique so far as the history of the medical corporations of Great Britain is concerned, was fulfilled for two centuries—that is until hospitals and dispensaries had become available to the sick poor.

FOR FURTHER READING

Clowes, W. *Selected Writings. Edited by F. N. L. Poynter.* 1948.
Comrie, J. D. *History of Scottish Medicine.* 2 vols. 1932.
Cushing, H. *A Bio-Bibliography of Andreas Vesalius.* New York. 1943.
Gnudi, M. T. and Webster, J. P. *The Life and Times of Gaspare Tagliacozzi, Surgeon of Bologna.* New York. 1950.
McMurrich, J. P. *Leonardo da Vinci the Anatomist.* Baltimore, 1930.
Packard, F. R. *The Life and Times of Ambroise Paré.* New York. 1926.
Paget, S. *Ambroise Paré and his Times.* 1897.
Parker, S. *The Early History of Surgery in Great Britain.* 1920.
Power, Sir D. *A Mirror for Surgeons.* Boston. 1939.
Power, Sir D. *Selected Writings.* 1931.
Singer, C. *The Evolution of Anatomy.* 1925.
South, J. F. *Memorials of the Craft of Surgery in England.* 1886.
Young, S. *The Annals of the Barber-Surgeons of London.* 1890.

CHAPTER SIX

The Seventeenth Century

No great advances in surgery were made in the early part of the seventeenth century. Amputation was still almost limited to cases of gangrene and it was performed by a circular method which differed little from one described by Celsus in the first century A.D. The means of arresting haemorrhage were still crude, difficult, and painful. John Woodall, one of the many prominent surgeons whose career spanned the end of the Tudor and the early part of the Stuart period, gives a graphic account of amputation by the circular method in his *Surgeon's Mate* of 1639.

"The amputation once resolved upon and all things ready for the work, let the Surgeon with all his assistances, and friends not forget before the beginning of the work heartily to call upon God for a blessing upon their endeavours, and let the patient the day before have notice given him that he also may take time to prepare himself with true resolution of soul and body to undergo the work, as being never performed without danger of death, which done, then let the Surgeon prepare himself also with his helpers, namely at the least five persons besides himself, as for example, one to sit behind the patient to hold him, a second for a holder, who by the surgeon must be instructed to stand fast before him and to bestride the limb to be amputated and to amplect [embrace] the limb; and a third to hold and stay the lower end of the diseased member to be taken off; a fourth to receive and bring back the sharp instruments; a fifth, to attend the Artist and deliver to him his needles and buttons, restrictive rollers, bolsters, bladder and so soon as possibly may be to stay with the palm of his hand the medicines applied to the end of the abscissed [amputated] stump that being the duty of the fifth helper and the sixth is the Artist himself that dismembereth. Six and not fewer are the least for the work of taking off a member proceeding by a wound by Gun-shot, done in the lacerated not totally mortified part. But for the taking off of a member in the mortified part three persons as assistants may serve, or two for the need, namely one to hold the upper part, the other the lower end. Let the surgeon have ready for instruments a fit amputating Cerra [saw], a Catlin [amputating knife], and a good small incision knife, a good pair of strong scissors and three or four cauterising instruments. Let one of the assistants take the upper part of the member, holding it in both hands reasonably fast and steady. I mean the whole part thereof somewhat near unto the unsound part and let the other helper hold the other part. I mean the putrid part to be abscissed in his hand whilst the Surgeon first by circumcising divide the putrid flesh from the bone doing it somewhat near the quick part but not too near it, about an inch full from the quick part that with the Cerra he may come without fear to divide the bone or bones asunder where he is sure they are sphacelated [gangrenous or mortified] not touching any quick part at all with his sharp instruments which he may observe the certainer to do, if with a Needle he enquire cautiously. Let him also divide betwixt the bones the parts there being lest by lacerating or tearing with the teeth of the Cerra he offend, which done let the Artist amputate the bones."

The first great advance on the old circular method of amputating came in 1679 through the advocacy of James Yonge, a naval surgeon of Plymouth. In that year Yonge published "A new way of amputation and a speedier convenient method of curing stumps than that commonly practised, in which (are) divers other useful matters recommended to the military Chirurgeon." Yonge acknowledged that he had obtained the first hint of the new method from another Devonshire surgeon, C. Lowdham, of Exeter. The manner of the operation was: "The Ligatures and Gripe [i.e. tourniquets and grip upon the limb by the assistants] being made after the common manner you are with your Catlin, or some long incision-knife, to raise (suppose it the Leg) a flap of the membranous flesh covering

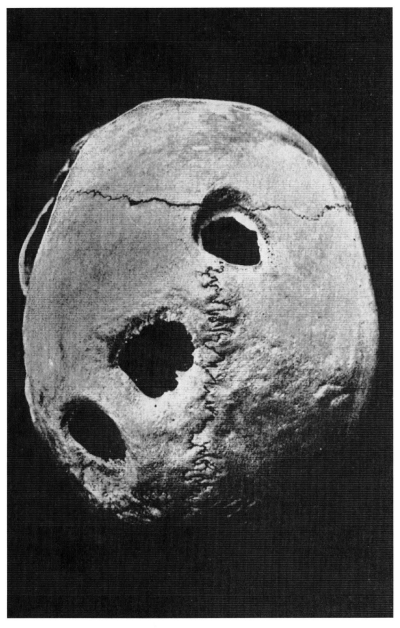

Pre-Columbian skull from Cuzco, Peru, showing three trephinations. It was not only possible but relatively easy to trephine a skull with a large flint. Many did survive the procedure, which was thought to be carried out as early as the New Stone Age

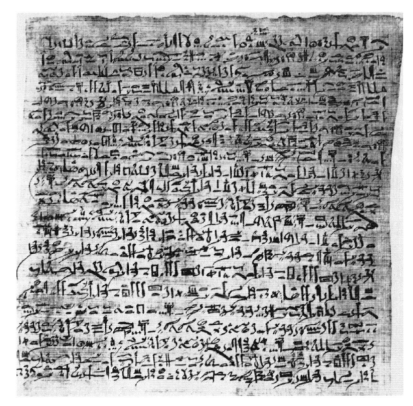

Case histories from the Edwin Smith Papyrus (1600 BC), the most ancient treatise. Acquired by the Egyptologist at Luxor in 1862. The knowledge and ideas they contain almost certainly relate to a considerably older period, perhaps five or six thousand years ago

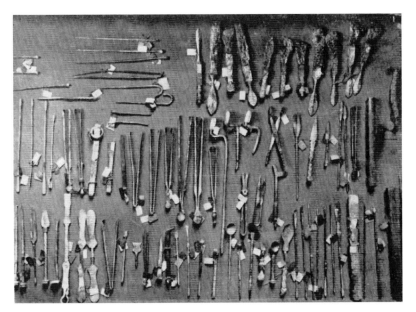

Roman surgical instruments found at Pompeii (1st century AD). The practice of medicine was considered to be beneath the dignity of Roman citizens and most of the medical and surgical practice of Rome was in the hands of Greeks

Arabic surgical instruments as illustrated in the writings of Abulcasis (AD 963-1013)

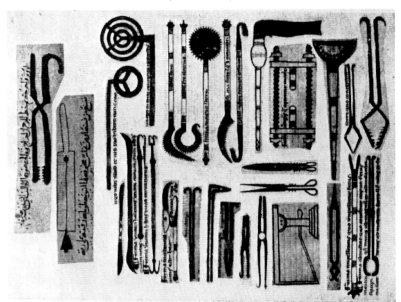

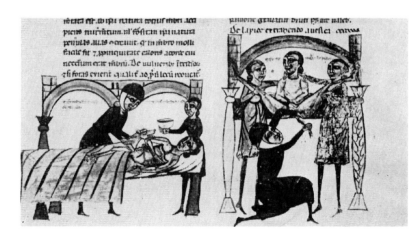

Surgical operations as depicted in a thirteenth-century manuscript of the Surgery of Roland of Parma. A nobleman of Bologna was so severely injured that a portion of his lung protruded through a wound. Roland boldly excised the protruding lung and the patient recovered well enough to later undertake a pilgrimage to Jerusalem

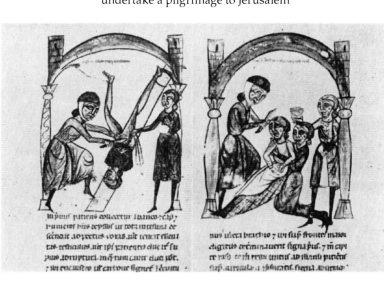

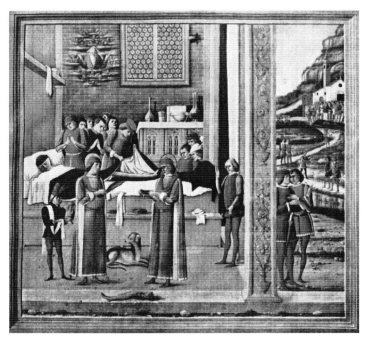

The miraculous amputation of a cancerous leg and its replacement
with the leg of a person who had just died, as performed by Saints
Cosmas and Damian. From a fifteenth-century miniature ascribed
to Andrea and Francesco Mantegna

An operation in the home. From the *Chirurgia* of Giovanni Andrea
della Croce, Venice, 1573

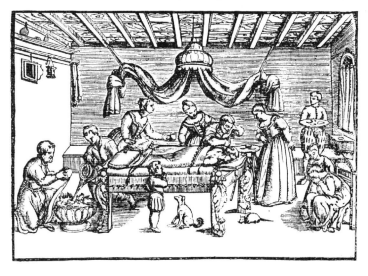

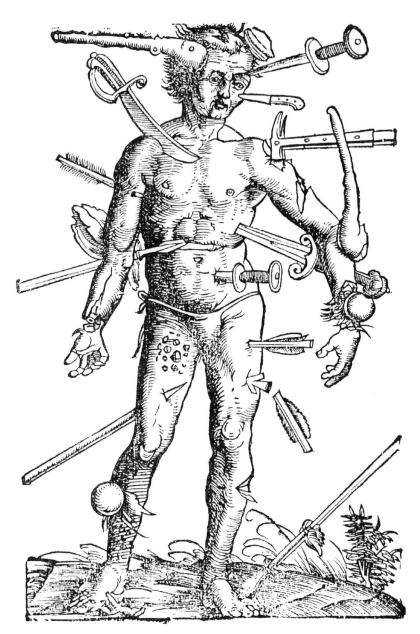

A Woundman, demonstrating the possible injuries a soldier could experience in battle. From Hans von Gersdorf's *Feldtbuch der Wundartznei*, Strassburg, 1530. Von Gersdorf had forty years' experience of campaigns and he produced a field book for the army surgeon. His work contains many striking illustrations of operation scenes, instruments and appliances

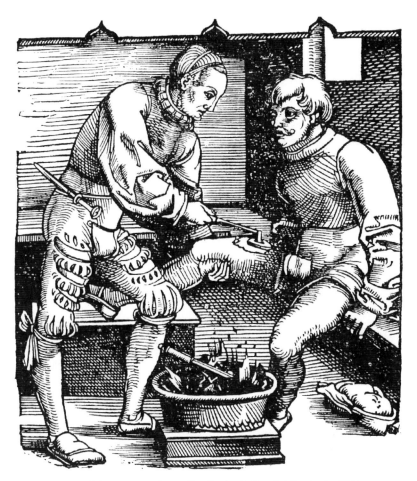

Use of the cautery. From Ibn Butlan's *Tacuini Sanitatis*, 1532

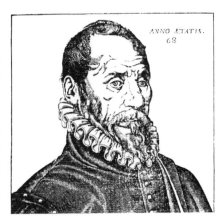

ANNO ÆTATIS.
68

Ambroise Paré (1510-90), the father of French surgery. The first man to break away from the old doctrine that 'diseases not curable by iron are curable by fire'. He became the greatest military surgeon of all time. He moved away from the practice of putting boiling oil into gunshot wounds after witnessing the suffering endured by patients

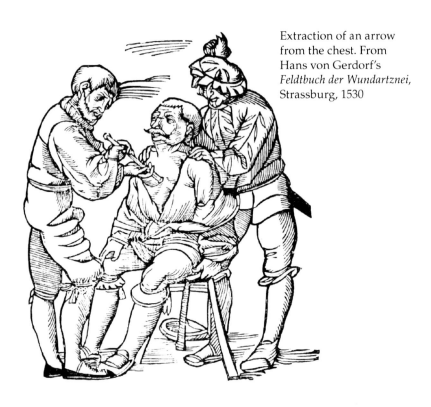

Extraction of an arrow
from the chest. From
Hans von Gerdorf's
Feldtbuch der Wundartznei,
Strassburg, 1530

A hospital ward in the sixteenth century. From the Great Surgery of
Paracelsus, Frankfurt, 1565

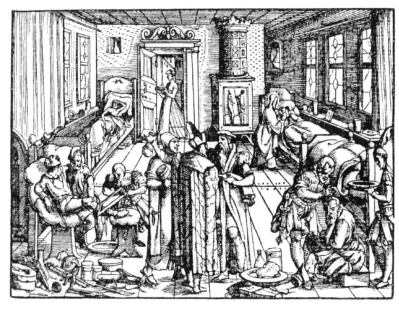

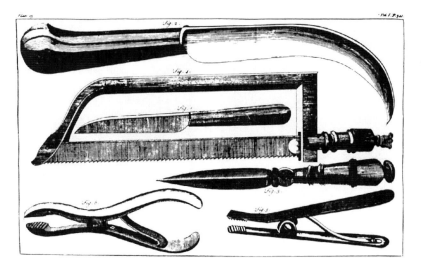

Amputation instruments from Lorenz Heister's *General System of Surgery*, 1753. Like nearly all great surgeons, he used few and simple instruments

Barron Larrey's flying ambulance, from a sketch by Duplessis-Bertaux in the Museum of Val de Grâce, Paris. Larrey went into the thick of battle to retrieve injured soldiers and administer aid to them more promptly

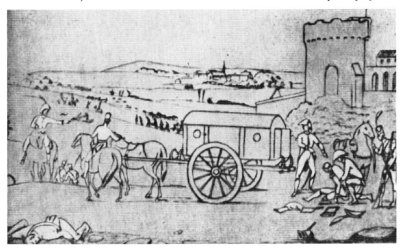

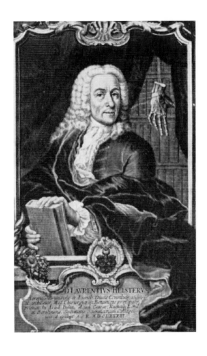

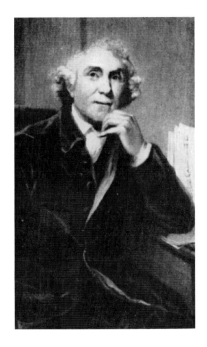

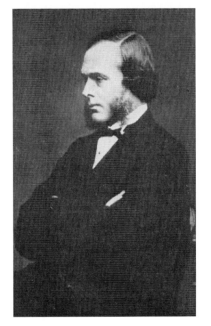

(Top left) Lorenz Heister
(1638–1758), great surgeon and
teacher of Helmstadt, Germany

(Top right) John Hunter (1728–93),
from an engraving by William
Sharp after the painting
by Sir Joshua Reynolds

(Left) Lord Lister (1827–1912),
from a photograph by T. & R.
Annan & Sons, Glasgow

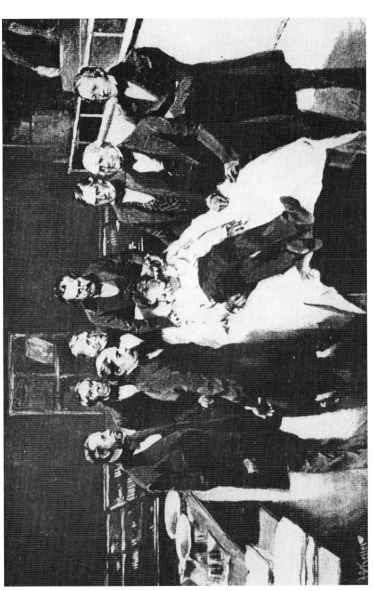

The first public demonstration of surgical anaesthesia, Massachusetts General Hospital, Boston, 16 October 1846. Its use rapidly spread to other parts of the world

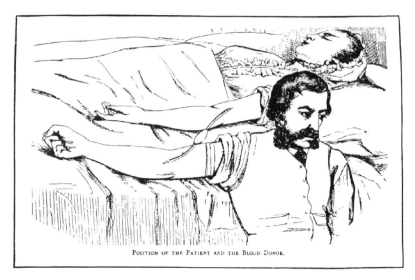

POSITION OF THE PATIENT AND THE BLOOD DONOR.

Direct blood transfusion in the treatment of haemorrhage following childbirth. After J.H. Aveling, 1873. The causes of many of the untoward effects of transfusion were not explained until 1901 when the presence of agglutinins and iso-agglutinins were demonstrated

Lister's carbolic spray in action. From Sir W. Watson Cheyne's *Antiseptic Surgery*, 1882. Lister's antiseptic ideas dramatically reduced death rates from sepsis where used

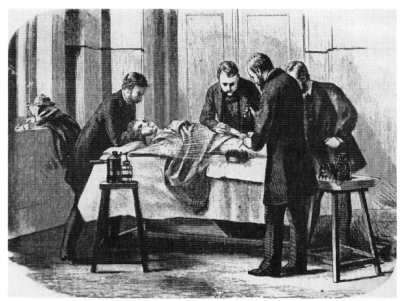

the muscles of the Calf, beginning below the place where you intend to make excision and raising it thitherward of length enought to cover the stump. Having so done turn it back under the hand of him that gripes; and, as soon as you have severed the member, bring this flap of cutaneous flesh over the stump and fasten it to the edges thereof by four or five strong stitches and, having so done, clap a dossil [plug] of lint into the inferior part, that one passage may be open for any blood or matter that may lodge between. Then lay on a common Defensative Ext. Bole, Sang. Dracon, Mastich, Terrae Sigil. cum alb. ovorum & Aceto and thereto gird it close with your cross bandage and other Compresses after the usual manner.''

The flap operation thus introduced soon came into use, although it underwent many modifications. The single flap was replaced by double flaps, and the method, at first restricted to the leg, was extended to the other limbs. In military practice, especially after gunshot and other shattering wounds, the circular method remained in favour.

James Yonge was a very remarkable man. Born in 1646 he was the son of John Yonge, a surgeon of Plymouth. After education at the local grammar school he was apprenticed to a naval surgeon, and he saw active service as a surgeon's mate in several ships, being present at the bombardment of Algiers in 1662 and having some extraordinary adventures. During a short interval on land he acted as assistant to an apothecary at Wapping and subsequently helped his father in practice at Plymouth. He then made voyages to Newfoundland and to the west coast of Africa. In 1665 his ship was captured by the Dutch and he was for nearly a year a prisoner at Amsterdam. He finally settled at Plymouth in 1670 and was appointed surgeon to the Naval Hospital at a salary of five shillings a day. In 1674 he was Deputy Surgeon-General of the Navy and in 1694 he was Mayor of Plymouth. In 1707 he embalmed the body of Sir Cloudesley Shovell, the Admiral who was drowned after his ship the *Association* had been wrecked on the Bishop Rock between Land's End and the Scilly Islands. Yonge died on 25 July, 1721, and was buried in St. Andrew's Church, Plymouth.

In 1633 appeared the earliest book on first-aid for the injured, the work of Dr. Stephen Bradwell. This was a small book with the very long title: *Helps for Suddain Accidents endangering life, by which those that live farre from Physicions or Chirurgions may happily preserve the life of a poore friend or neighbour till such a man may be had to perfect the cure.* On the whole the advice given does not seem to be very practical and in some cases the measures proposed would appear very odd to a modern first-aider. Thus the cure for the "Biting of a Madde Dogge" is to throw the patient into water. "In doing this, if he cannot swim, after he hath swallowed a good quantity of water, take him out again. But if he be skilful in swimming, hold him under the water a little while till he have taken in some pretty quantity."

The outstanding surgeon of seventeenth-century England was Richard Wiseman (1622–76), surgeon to James I and Charles II. He was for a time a surgeon in the Navy and he then served with the army of Charles I until the final defeat by Cromwell at Worcester in 1651. Then followed a period of service with the Spanish Navy. At the Restoration Wiseman returned to London and was appointed surgeon to Charles II. His book *Several Chirurgical Treatises*, published in the year of his death, was the greatest work on surgery which had appeared in English up to that time. One of Wiseman's duties as royal surgeon was to examine patients coming to be "touched" by the king for the king's evil, i.e. tuberculosis of the lymph glands of the neck. This malady, also known as scrofula, was very common. The power of curing the disease by touch had been attributed to anointed kings from early times although the first English king to treat the evil was Edward the Confessor. The custom reached its zenith during the Stuart period and it is stated that Charles II actually touched on an average four thousand persons every year. The cure was attended by great ceremony and there was a special service incorporated into the Prayer Book. Each patient received a gold coin or "touch piece" and it has been well remarked that "Some were cured of the king's evil, who never had any other evil than that of poverty, which brought more patients and more fame to those royal practitioners than they deserved." Or as another wit put it, "What the sovereign could not cure, the half sovereign could." Even during his exile in Holland Charles II was so besieged by sufferers seeking relief that on one occasion six people were trampled to death. William of Orange was sceptical of the royal power for he touched but few, saying, "God grant you better health and more sense." Wiseman gives an excellent account of the king's evil and states, "I have myself been an eye witness of hundreds of cures performed by his Majesty's touch alone, without any assistance of chirurgery." Nevertheless he shows what surgery can do when the king is not available.

Wiseman gives a graphic account of gunshot wounds, describing many cases from his vast experience. The following report dates from the period when he was serving at sea:

"Whilst our squadron rode at anchor in the Groin, there came in some Hollanders, under the notion of Hamburgers, with three ships new trimmed up for the King of Spain's service. A boatswain of one of these ships happened in company ashore with some of our men, where drinking together, the Hollander began to prate of religion, upbraiding one of our men for wearing a cross; and after a while, growing more heated with drink, he became quarrelsome and swore sacrement he would not wear a cross, no, the Devil take him, repeating it often. One of our men beat him down and fell with him; then kneeling upon his breast and holding his head down, he drew out a knife sticking in his sash and cut him from the eye towards the mouth then from the os zygoma to the netherjaw. Now, said he, you shall wear a cross that the Devil do not carry you away. I was sent for from the next house and stitched the lips of the wounds close together, then sprinkling them with a little pulv. Galeni, applied pledgets with sarcotick ungent, and with astringents and bandage dressed him. The next morning he was let blood and the third day I took off the dressings, and finding the wound as it were agglutinated in the slits, I cut out some of the stitches, sprinkled the wound as at first and dressed him up with sarcoticks, with compress and bandage. The second day after I dresssed him again and cut out the remaining stitches; and in a dressing or two cured him. This being the work of Nature, who rarely faileth in acting her part if we perform ours, in retaining the lips close together and defending them from fluxion. The patient was well pleased with his cure, though there remained some marks of a cross, these sort of people wearing them with much pride in their faces, as marks of their courage."

This story of an accident illustrates one of the perils of life in the seventeenth century:

"A gentleman of about thirty years of age coming out of Hertfordshire through Tottenham and riding upon the causeway near an inn, one emptying a chamber pot out of the window as he was passing by, his horse started and rushed violently between a signpost and a tree which supported part of the sign. The poor gentleman was beaten off his horse and lay stunned on the ground."

A barber-surgeon was hastily summoned but nothing much was done for the injured man until Wiseman arrived.

"I found the gentleman lying upon the ground, the people and chirurgeon gazing upon him. I felt his pulse much opressed, the right brow bruised and inquired whether they had bled him blood. The chirurgeon replied he had opened a vein in his arm but it would not bleed. I replied, we must make him bleed through it by splitting his veins. Turning his head on one side, I saw the jugular vein on the bruised side turgid and opened it. He bled freely. After I had taken about twelve ounces, the blood ran down from his arm which had been opened before and would not bleed. We bled him till he came to life, and then he raved and struggled with us."

The patient's injuries were dressed and he was subjected to further bleedings but made a good recovery.

Wiseman had great experience of gunshot wounds. He rejected the idea that they were venomous but was well aware of the danger of retained foreign bodies, particularly pieces of clothing. Here is a typical case:

"The servant of a nobleman was wounded and shot in

the thigh by highwaymen. The bullet not being extracted by his country chirurgeon at the first dressing, could not be drawn out by me at the second, but occasioned great pain and inflammation, burning heat and watchings. And although he had many other considerable wounds upon him to make a derivation, yet was his gunshot more vexatious than all the rest, until I extracted the bullet and rags carried with it: yet this was but a pistol bullet. But after I had drawn it out, my digestion [i.e. suppuration] became good; and by equal bandage, with gentle compression of the parts, I united and healed it in ten or twelve days, which I doubt would not have been cured in three months."

Wiseman was well acquainted with the bizarre results of some gunshot wounds. He refers to a case in which a bullet entered the cheek and was extracted from the back of the neck and another in which a missile entering the arm was removed from below the shoulder blade.

He stresses the need for a quick amputation if it is to be done at all, if only for the reason that operations performed in the heat of a fight are easier for the patient to bear. Once in the middle of a naval battle he cut off a man's arm and immediately after, as the fight grew hotter, the man got up and ran to help traverse a gun.

Fireworks were a frequent cause of accidents then as now, as the following case from Wiseman's book shows:

"A young gentleman of about ten years of age boarded at a school a few miles off, the evening before the fifth of November having filled his right pocket full of squibs and crackers, threw one of them into the chimney amongst the embers. It took fire, but whether it scattered the fire and some spark of that flew into his pocket, or whether it was the cracker, but those in his pocket took fire also and his clothes burnt. At the sight whereof his little chamber-fellow ran out for help. In his absence a little boy from some other apartment took the alarm, came in, and seeing his school fellow in a flame, catched up a basin of water and threw it upon him, then ran away for help. Others came in and rescued him out of his burnt clothes. A neighbouring chirurgeon was sent for, who dressed him."

The next day the boy was brought to Wiseman. He had burns on the right side extending from the armpit to the knee and his hand and arm were also burnt from his efforts to pull the burning fireworks from his pocket. He was dressed with fine lawn dipped in oil of bitter almonds, oil of elders, egg yolks, stramonium and other substances and was completely healed.

Wiseman makes frequent reference to two methods of treatment which were very much employed by surgeons in the seventeenth century—issues (also known as fontanells) and setons. An issue was a small ulcer made by means of a red hot iron, lancet, scissors or by the application of some corrosive substance with the idea of providing for the expulsion of morbid matter. Issues were commonly made at the back of the neck, in the arm, or below the knee. The ulcer so produced was kept open by the insertion of a foreign body, such as a pill of gold or silver, lint, wax, orris root, or very commonly a pea.

The seton was a special kind of issue made by drawing a strip of silk or linen through a wound made in the skin. As described by William Salmon in his *Ars Chirurgica* (1699) the technique was as follows:

"Take up the skin with a perforated pair of forceps, nip it pretty hard to stupify it. Through the perforations of the forceps and skin, pass a needle red hot, after which, with another needle, bring through the silken string or cord. Afterwards let the string be drawn every day sometimes to this side, sometimes to that, that the mattery part may hang out of the wound: the ulcer is thus to be kept open, as long as need requires." The idea behind these drastic methods of treatment, as with the universal practice of blood-letting, was to "evacuate superfluous humours". In the same way, as suppuration was regarded as an inevitable consequence of almost any wound, wounds were deliberately kept open to provide for the exit of pus. A favourite method, and one used by all the surgeons of the sixteenth and seventeenth centuries, was by the insertion of "tents" into the wound; these were bunches or rolls of linen or other material. One other peculiar therapeutic measure remains to be mentioned. This was moxibustion, a method introduced into European medicine in the seventeenth century from the Far East by William ten Rhyne, a Dutch physician. Moxa is the soft down collected from the dried leaves of the plant Mugwort (*Artemesia vulgaris*). This material was made into little cones which were placed on the skin and then ignited. Moxibustion was, like that other favourite Chinese method of treatment acupuncture, a means of producing counter-irritation.

Superstition was rife in the seventeenth century; it was a great time for witch-hunting, and alongside the skilful and rational treatment of surgeons like Wiseman there were other methods based on the most absurd superstitions. One of the most extraordinary beliefs was that there is a "sympathy" existing between certain inanimate objects, such as articles of clothing and their owner and between a wound and the weapon that inflicted the wound. This superstition took many forms. Reference has already been made to the case related by Ambroise Paré in which a charlatan claimed to be able to cure a fractured leg by means of the patient's girdle. The idea was that as the girdle was fastened to form an unbroken ring so would the leg mend and become whole. A curious manifestation of this belief in sympathetic magic was the widespread use of the weapon salve. The weapon salve or ointment was applied not to the wound but to the weapon that caused the wound. This was the method of treatment adopted by the Lady Margaret when she found William of Deloraine grievously wounded and with a broken lance still in his side, as told by Sir Walter Scott in *The Lay of the Last Minstrel.*

> "She drew the splinter from the wound,
>   And with a charm she stanched the blood;
>   She bade the gash be cleansed and bound:
>   No longer by his couch she stood;
>   But she has ta'en the broken lance,
>   And washed it from the clotted gore,
>   And salved the splinter o'er and o'er."

The idea of the sympathetic ointment is attributed to that

extraordinary figure, Paracelsus (1490–1541), who was long regarded as a charlatan but is now acknowledged to have been one of the most original medical thinkers of his time.

"Take moss growing on a skull exposed to the weather, and of human fat each two ounces, of mummy and human blood each half an ounce, oil or roses, bole armeniac each one ounce, linseed oil two draghms. Make an ointment and preserve it in a box. When you have to treat a wound simply dip a splinter of wood in the blood and when dry stick the wood in the ointment. Bandage the wound every morning with a new cloth soaked in the patient's urine. So it will heal without any other application, and you may thus cure a patient ten or twenty miles off, if you only have his blood. Also if you have a weapon with which a man has been wounded and annoint it with a certain ointment, the wound will heal without pain."

In spite of attacks this superstition flourished and even so excellent a surgeon as Fabricius Hildanus was disposed to believe in it: "In 1613 the Lady Anna Sidonia Bremserina of Rüdesherm on the Rhine having happily recovered from childbirth was somehow wounded in the left breast by a knife. Her friends, leaving the wound to itself, diligently anointed and bandaged the knife. The wound healed rapidly on the surface, but was followed by an abscess and severe febrile symptoms, which so frightened her relations that they sent for me." Fabricius treated the abscess by free incision and she recovered. In this case he observes the weapon salve may have said to have failed but he explains the failure by saying that it was generally believed to have been revealed to Paracelsus by the devil, and the patient was a lady of such singular piety that nothing devilish could have any effect on her."

Fabricius Hildanus (1560–1634) was city surgeon at Berne where he also kept a private hospital and gave clinical instruction. He had a large museum and was skilful in inventing new instruments such as aural specula, splints, and forceps for removing foreign bodies. His chief work was entitled *Six-hundred Surgical Cures and Observations*. The following is one of his case histories dated 25 April, 1624:

"A countryman, Benedict Barquin bought some iron and was striking two pieces together to prove its quality, when a splinter flew into his eye and stuck in the cornea, causing him great pain. The local surgeons tried everything for many days to no purpose, and the pain and inflammation so increased that he came to me at Berne on 5th March. I used all means I could think of for some days, but the splinter was so small that it could not be removed by instruments. When behold! My wife hit on the very thing. I kept the eye open with both hands, while she held a magnet as close as possible to it, and after several trials (for he could not stand the necessary light long), we saw the iron leap from the eye to the stone."

This ingenious lady was a great help to her husband and we are told that in his absence she was capable of treating not only the diseases of her own sex but even cases of fractured ribs and legs.

Fabricius also tells the story of a modest and pious maiden named Susanna who fell into the hands of the soldiers when the Duke of Savoy waged war against Geneva in 1590. They cut off her nose. Two years later John Griffonius, an ingenious surgeon, came to Lausanne and undertook to make her a new nose which he did to the greatest admiration of all men. "I myself," writes Fabricius, "have often seen and examined it. The nose has undergone no change and the marks of operation are hardly visible; but in winter when it is very cold the tip turns a little blue."

Fabricius is probably most widely known through his method of amputating with a red-hot knife. This plan had been used, or at least recommended, by Arabic and medieval surgeons, but Fabricius improved it, as he considered, by increasing the thickness of the instrument, so that it could retain the heat throughout the operation. The method has, he declares, three great advantages: (1) it is less painful; (2) the muscles are more completely retracted, and therefore the bone may be divided higher up; (3) the loss of blood is very much less than when either a separate cautery or ligature is employed; and he narrates how, by means of this hot knife he successfully amputated the leg above the knee, in a patient attacked by gangrene following dysentery, who was so prostrated that even a moderate loss of blood would have been fatal.

Johann Schultz (Scultetus) of Ulm (1595–1645) distinguished himself by his ingenuity in devising artificial limbs, eyes, noses and surgical instruments. He left many observations which throw light upon the practice of his time. He was a bold operator even in his younger days. "While I was studying medicine in Padua, a noble undergraduate suffered for some months from a swelling of his left hand, which was not benefited by general or local treatment, and began to ulcerate in the palm. So we consulted the illustrious Spigelius who, putting a probe in the ulcer, reached carious bone, and said it was spina ventosa, an incurable disease, which attacks bones first and corrodes them without affecting the periosteum, or causing pain; then it forms a slightly painful swelling, and after some months the part ulcerates. I obtained permission of the patient and amputated his hand below the carpus."

The chief Italian surgeons of the century were Pietro de Marchetti (1589–1675) professor at Padua, and Marcus Aurelius Severinus of Naples (1580–1656). There was at this time an exaggerated idea as to the danger of suturing divided tendons, a dread which was not removed until the famous Swiss Albrecht von Haller carried out experiments on animals in the following century. Marchetti wrote: "Nerves and tendons must never be sutured, for this practice is often followed by fatal tetanus. The ingenious surgeon should rather remedy deformities by appropriate splints, as I did in the case of a distinguished Marshal of France, of the family of Montmorency. He received a sword cut on the right wrist, dividing the extensor tendons of the thumb. When the wound healed the thumb was drawn across the palm of the hand, so that he could not hold sword, dagger or lance, and was entirely incapacitated for the profession of arms, apart from which he declared life was not worth living. So he consulted me about amputating his hand, to which I could in no wise consent, but divised an iron case to hold the thumb out, fixed by two cords to bracelets round the wrist, and so he was able to hold and use all kinds of weapons."

Marchetti also gives an account of a case of traumatic epilepsy cured by trephining. "I was once called in consultation with doctor Julius Sala, professor at Padua, to a patient who had been struck on the head with a dagger, with lesion of the skull, membranes, and brain itself. The wound healed externally, but was followed in three or four months by recurrent epileptic attacks. On introducing a probe I found the above mentioned penetrating wound. I therefore enlarged the opening with a trephine, letting out much yellow ichor, and in thirty days both the wound and the epilepsy were completely cured."

There are very few early accounts of operations for the removal of tumours. Cancer of the breast was occasionally treated by excision, by the cautery, or by the application of caustics, as were small external growths and excrescences. Nothing beyond general palliative measures could be done for a patient suffering from an internal cancer. The contemporary record of an operation performed in 1665 for removal of a fatty tumour from a German soldier is therefore of special interest. This is how Dr. John Sigismund Elsholtz, of Berlin, describes the case:

"Michael Nebel, a Captain of the Foot Guards of his Serene Highness our Elector, consulted me in the autumn of the year 1665. He said that six years ago he noticed a lump, no bigger than a pea, near the perinaeum on the border of the nates close to the anus.

"He had not taken advice because it caused no pain or trouble but it had increased in size until it extended to the front of the left groin. It had become so big in the course of the last month that the skin had first stretched and then given way and during the last few days it had grown still more rapidly. The patient, who was thirty-seven years of age, tall, thin and healthy, said further that the only inconvenience the swelling had caused him was formerly when he was a dragoon and had to ride, and he dated the beginning of the swelling from that time.

"The swelling felt hard and was so resilient on pressure that it seemed at first sight to be a sarcoma or fleshy tumour. He

was advised to have it removed piecemeal as it might sup-
purate, but as he did not agree to this it was decided to
remove it at one sitting. The operation was fixed for December 6th and the patient was ordered to be purged and bled
in preparation for it. About eight o'clock in the morning
Dr. Martin Weise, junior, and I as the physicians, with two
surgeons were in attendance and when everything was
ready the patient was laid upon the operating table. He
declined to be tied down as he thought it was unbecoming
for a soldier, but nevertheless we had two lusty men who held
his arms and legs. The tumour was first wrapped in lint on
account of its slipperiness and its base was transfixed with
a needle and thread from one side and then with a second
needle and thread from the other side. The ligatures were
tied tightly in case there might be severe bleeding. The
whole mass was then cut away quickly with a sharp knife,
and a dressing soaked in white of egg and bole was applied
at once to the wound. The leg was then bandaged and for
greater security a bandage was put round the belly, and the
patient who had borne the operation manfully was put
back to bed.

"Twenty-four hours later the tighter bandages were
removed and the others were loosened but the styptic
dressing was left untouched. Appropriate remedies were
given from time to time and the wound healed in a month."

Dr. Elsholtz, the physician who recorded this case, was one
of the first, after the English pioneers Wren and Lower, to
carry out experiments on blood transfusion and was the author
of one of the earliest books on transfusion in 1667. It will be
noted that the name of the surgeon who actually performed
the operation is not even mentioned in the case record. This
is entirely in accord with the two branches of the medical
profession at the time: the surgeon was regarded as being
quite inferior to the physician and in what was for that time
a major operation, could only act under his authority. In
England at the same period it was laid down that "no surgeon
be so bold as to trepan, or open the belly except in the presence
and on the advice of a physician." The tumour weighed two

pounds, and in view of the difficulty of controlling haemorrhage in such a case its successful removal was a great feat. But if credit is due to the operator, what can we say of the courage of the patient who refused to be tied down because "it was not becoming to a soldier"?

Although the seventeenth century was not marked by any revolutionary advances in surgery some surgeons became very skilful. Considering the limitations imposed by the imperfect knowledge of their time and particularly the absence of any means of preventing pain and sepsis, we cannot but admire their achievements.

The ailments of famous people have always excited interest and there are records of some very notable operations carried out on great figures of history. During the seventeenth century stone in the bladder continued to be one of the most prevalent diseases. Samuel Pepys, the diarist, was cut for stone on 26 March, 1658, and unfortunately from the medical point of view this was two years before he began to write his Diary. He decided to keep the anniversary of his deliverance as a festival, and on 26 March, 1660, he wrote: "This day is two years since it pleased God that I was cut for the stone at Mrs. Turner's in Salisbury Court. And did resolve while I live to keep it as a festival, as I did the last year at my house and for ever to have Mrs. Turner and her company with me." Mrs. Turner was a relative of Pepys and she lived next door to his father, who had a tailor's shop in Salisbury Court, Fleet Street. It was usual at this period to arrange for surgical operations to be performed in the house of a friend or quite often at an inn; a private patient of means would not have been admitted to a hospital and there were no nursing homes in those days.

The man who operated on Pepys was Thomas Hollyer, surgeon to St. Thomas's Hospital and an expert lithotomist. In one year he cut thirty patients for stone, all of whom lived; his next four patients all died. Such runs or unsuccessful cases are encountered by nearly all surgeons of large practice even in the present day, and apart from the fact that every major operation carries a certain incalculable element of risk, they may be explained by the fact that the patients concerned may have been suffering from other infirmities—were in fact "bad risks".

In pre-antiseptic days, however, such runs of disaster were sometimes accounted for by the presence of infection in the hospital or by the fact that the surgeon may have allowed his instruments to become septic. However this may be, Samuel Pepys was delivered from the torment of his stone and made a good recovery. Unfortunately—and this was a not uncommon sequel of the operation at the time—his spermatic ducts were injured at the time of operation and although, as every reader of his Diary knows, this did not lessen his sexual urge, it made him sterile.

Pepys was led by his personal experience and his natural curiosity to take a lively interest in things medical. On 27 February, 1662, he records a visit to the Hall of the Barber-Surgeons' Company in Monkwell Street:

"Up and to my office, whither several persons came to me about office business. About 11 o'clock Commissioner Pett and I walked to Chirurgeon's Hall (we being all invited thither and promised to dine there); where we were led into the Theatre; and by and by comes the reader, Dr. Tearne, with the Master and Company, in a very handsome manner; and all being settled, he began his lecture, this being the second upon the kidneys, ureters, &c. which was very fine; and his discourse being ended, we walked into the Hall, and there being great store of company, we had a fine dinner and good learned company, many Doctors of Phisique, and we used with extraordinary great respect. After dinner Dr. Scarborough took some of his friends and I went along with them, to see the body alone, which we did, which was a lusty fellow, a seaman that was hanged for a robbery. I did touch the body with my bare hand; it felt cold, but methought it was a very unpleasant sight. Thence we went into a private room where I perceive they prepare the bodies, and there were the kidneys, ureters, &c. upon which he read to-day, and Dr. Scarborough upon my desire and the company's did show very clearly the manner of the disease of the stone and the cutting and all other questions that I could think of. . . . Thence, with great satisfaction to me, back to the Company, where I heard good discourse, and so to the afternoon Lecture upon the heart and lungs, &c. and that being done we broke up, took leave and back to the office."

As we have seen, the Barber-Surgeons' Company had the right to claim four bodies annually of persons executed for felony, and it was one of the Anatomy lectures illustrated by the dissection of such a body that Pepys attended. At this period there was nothing unusual in the presence of a distinguished civil servant such as Pepys, who was moreover a Fellow of the Royal Society and an intimate friend of some of the most distinguished medical men of the day, at such a gruesome performance. Anatomy lectures, both in this country and abroad, long continued to have much of the character of a public spectacle.

An even more notable patient than Pepys was Louis XIV of France, who suffered for many years from that very painful and undignified condition, anal fistula. In 1686 the King was operated upon by one of his surgeons, C. F. Felix, with complete success. The operation took place at seven o'clock in the morning and it says much for the stoicism of the King that he insisted on holding his levee at the accustomed hour of eight. He behaved with great courage throughout the operation and continually encouraged the surgeon in his nerve-racking task. Felix, who was already receiving a salary of about £1,200 a year, was rewarded with a fee of £15,000, a country estate and a patent of nobility. A remarkable result of the operation was that Felix was inundated by requests from courtiers who entreated him to perform the same operation upon them. Those who were told that the surgeon saw not the faintest reason for complying with their demand were greatly annoyed, while it is recorded that the few sycophants who really suffered from anal fistula "could not contain their pride and joy". Felix's success brought about a revolution in the status of French surgeons. Before his time the organization of surgical practice in France was similar to that in England. There was a College of St. Côme founded about 1210 and consisting of real surgeons (surgeons of the long robe), and there was also a guild of barber-surgeons (surgeons of the short robe). These two corporations constantly quarrelled with each other and with the Faculty of Medicine. In general the status of the surgeon was very low, but thanks to the prestige won by Felix and to the efforts of Georges Maréschal, another surgeon to Louis XIV, surgery was recognized as a liberal art and its exponents were accorded a much higher rank in society.

In the sixteenth century surgeons began to be provided with reliable guides to human anatomy. The seventeenth century saw the rise of experimental physiology, a science to which Englishmen made contributions of the greatest significance for the future progress of medicine and surgery. The greatest event of all was the discovery of the circulation of the blood. That the blood was in motion had been known from the earliest times but up to the seventeenth century it had been supposed that it ebbed to and fro like the tides. No one had any real idea as to the function of the blood but some thought that it served to cool the body. One or two investigators had arrived at an inkling of the fact that the blood circulates but definite proof of this was first given by Dr. William Harvey, physician to St. Bartholomew's Hospital and to Charles I in 1628. Harvey showed by means of experiments and careful measurement that the heart acts as a pump and propels the blood round the body in a continuous cycle or circle. From the immediate practical point of view knowledge of the way in which the blood circulated proved of immense benefit to medicine and surgery. One thing that Harvey's theory did was to provide a rational basis for the practice of blood transfusion and for intravenous medication.

The vital importance of the blood must have been appreciated from the dawn of human history. It was invested with all kinds of properties, spiritual as well as physical. Drinking the blood of enemies or of wild beasts was supposed to confer vigour.

Vague references to the transfusion of blood are found in old writers, but medical men were obsessed with the idea of taking blood out of the body rather than putting it in. There is a story that an attempt was made about the year 1490 to prolong the life of Pope Innocent VIII by means of a blood transfusion. According to one account, a Jewish physician transfused the aged Pontiff with blood from three small boys, who were each to receive a ducat as a reward. Another source states that the blood was given in the form of a draught. The testimony is conflicting and there is no proof that the Pope received either the transfusion or the drink. One of the earliest proposals for the transfusion of blood was made by Andreas Libavius, a physician of Halle in Saxony, in 1615. In 1628, the very year of the publication of Harvey's book on the circulation, Giovanni Colle, professor of medicine at Padua, suggested that blood could be transfused but he certainly never carried out the experiment. Another Italian physician, Francesco Folli, in 1680 advised transfusion by the insertion of a silver tube into the artery of the donor and a bone cannula in the vein of the recipient, uniting the two by means of a tube. He gave a full description of the apparatus required and suggested that twenty young men should act as blood donors, but he confessed that he had not attempted to carry his idea into practice. Francis Potter, an eccentric English clergyman, had the idea of curing diseases by blood transfusion as early as 1640 and carried out some experiments on hens. He attempted to collect blood from a vein in the leg by means of an ivory pipe and a bladder, but found that he could only procure two or three drops.

The first serious attempts at blood transfusion were made in England and France. As early as 1657 that great genius, Sir Christopher Wren, carried out numerous experiments on the injection of liquids into the veins of animals. In one experiment he made a dog drunk by injecting wine and beer into its veins. Wren was one of the founders of the Royal Society, and in 1667 it was stated with reference to his work, "Hence arose many new experiments, and chiefly that of transfusing blood, which the Society has prosecuted in sundry instances, that will probably end in extraordinary success."

In 1665 Dr. Richard Lower of Oxford carried out successful transfusion from artery to vein in dogs. He at first used quills for uniting the blood vessels of the two dogs, but afterwards found that silver tubes connected by a piece of the cervical artery of an ox were more satisfactory. This is the first definite record of transfusion of blood from one animal to another. Similar experiments on transfusion in animals were carried out about a year later by Jean Denys, a professor in the medical faculty of Paris. These experiments proved that an animal that had been rendered moribund by bleeding could be restored to full health by a transfusion, and their success led Denys to take the further step of attempting to transfuse the blood of one kind of animal into the veins of another kind. In March 1667 the blood of a calf was transfused into the veins of a dog, apparently without ill effect. Then came the crucial experiment. On 15 June, 1667, Denys transfused a youth of fifteen who had been suffering from a fever, for which he had been bled so many times that "his wit seemed wholly sunk, his memory perfectly lost, and his body so heavy and drowsy that he was not fit for anything". A further three ounces of blood was taken from the lad and he received in exchange about nine ounces from the carotid artery of a lamb. The patient was greatly improved and the only ill effect he experienced was a feeling of great heat along his arm. Denys carried out a second successful transfusion upon an old man, but some of his later patients were not so lucky. One man who received the blood of a calf showed all the signs of receiving incompatible blood and was very fortunate to escape with his life.

Meanwhile the Royal Society group had also carried their experiments to the point where they were ready to transfuse human beings. On 23 November, 1667, Drs. Richard Lower and Edmund King successfully transfused the blood of a sheep into Arthur Coga, a Bachelor of Divinity of Cambridge, aged thirty-two. A few days later Samuel Pepys, who was one of the original Fellows of the Royal Society, met the subject of this experiment at a dinner party, and he recorded in his famous Diary: "I was pleased to see the person who had his blood taken out. He speaks well, and did this day give the Society a relation thereof in Latin, saying that he finds himself much better since, and as a new man, but he is cracked a little in his head, though he speaks very reasonably and very well. He had but 20s. for his suffering it, and is to have the same again tried upon him: the first sound man that ever had it tried upon him in England, and but one that we hear of in France, which was a porter hired by the virtuosoes."

In 1668 one of Denys's patients died after the third of a series of transfusions and the widow instituted proceedings against him. The case aroused great feeling and a verdict was given against Denys. It was directed that in future no transfusion was to be performed without the permission of the Faculty of Medicine of Paris. As the Faculty was bitterly opposed to the whole idea, permission was never given, and in 1670 the practice of transfusion was forbidden by law. This disaster had its repercussions in London. The records of the Royal Society show that poor cracked-brained Arthur Coga did have a second transfusion without any serious effect on 14 December, 1667, and it appears that a few further animal experiments were made in 1669. After that no more was heard of blood transfusion in England for more than a hundred years. What the pioneers of transfusion did not know was that animal blood contains proteins that are totally incompatible with those in human blood. In attempting transfusion from man to man they were unable to overcome the technical difficulties connected with clotting and they knew nothing about the blood groups. Nevertheless they did enough to show that blood transfusion could be a means of saving life.

FOR FURTHER READING

Crawfurd, R. *The King's Evil.* 1911.

Degueret, E. *Histoire Médicale du Grand Roi (Louis XIV).* Paris. 1924.

Guthrie, D. *A History of Medicine.* 1945.

Keynes, G. *Blood Transfusion.* Bristol. 1949.

Lindeboom, G. A. The story of a blood transfusion to a Pope. *J. Hist. Med.,* 1954, *9,* 455.

Longmore, Sir T. *Richard Wiseman, a Biographical Study.* 1891.

Maluf, N. S. R. History of blood transfusion. *J. Hist. Med.,* 1954, *9,* 59.

Power, Sir D. The brave soldier: an operation for the removal of a fatty tumour in the year 1665. *Med. J. & Rec., N.Y.,* 1926, *123,* 258.

Power, Sir D. An historical lithotomy: Mr. Samuel Pepys. *Brit. J. Surg.,* 1931, *18,* 541.

Shelley, H. S. Cutting for the stone. *J. Hist. Med.,* 1958, *13,* 50.

Zimmerman, L. and Howell, K. M. History of blood transfusion. *Ann. med. Hist.,* 1932, N. S. *4,* 415.

CHAPTER SEVEN

The Eighteenth Century

FRENCH surgeons took a prominent part in the advancement of surgery during the eighteenth century. In the early part of the century the greatest names were those of Dominique Anel, Jean Louis Petit, and in the second half Pierre Desault and François Chopart. Anel joined the Army in early youth and attained the rank of surgeon-major. He gives an interesting sketch of military surgery during the wars of Louis XIV. Educated surgeons were few, their place being supplied by "wound suckers", some of whom were old soldiers but others had never served and were entirely ignorant of surgery. They all pretended to cure wounds by sucking them, after which they poured in a little oil, muttering certain charms, and then covered the whole with a compress. The charms, says Anel, are nonsense; the oil does neither harm nor good; sucking is sometimes of great use in removing blood clots and foreign bodies which prevent direct union. But as it was disgusting and dangerous to do this with the mouth, Anel invented an ingenious suction syringe. Another of his achievements was the well-known operation of curing aneurysm by ligature of the artery immediately above the sac, which he successfully performed on a monk at Rouen in 1710. Three years later he was the first to pass a probe through the tear duct of a living being, and he invented a minute syringe to inject fluids into the sac; by this means he was able to cure cases of lachrymal abscess without the use of knife or cautery.

J. L. Petit also began as an army surgeon, and his military experiences no doubt helped him in the invention of the famous screw tourniquet. He improved the circular method of amputation by dividing the soft parts in two incisions instead of one, and he pointed out the great importance of removing all suspicious glands in operations for cancer. He was also the first to perform a successful operation for mastoiditis. Finally he became director of the Royal Academy of Surgery, which had been established in 1731. This body did a great deal to improve surgery and to raise the status of the surgeon in France.

The name of Pierre Desault is connected with a bandage for fractured collar-bone, but an even more important service he rendered was the introduction of the gum-elastic catheter. He also introduced the straight amputating knife, and the modern form of wire snare or *écraseur*. His greatest contribution was probably the development of clinical instruction in surgery, in which he was aided by his friend François Chopart, well known for his operation on the foot—Chopart's amputation.

France had many other distinguished surgeons at this time. Augustin Belloste and François de la Peyronie made important observations on head injuries. Antoine Louis, secretary of the Royal Academy of Surgery, was a noted surgeon and anatomist who also wrote on the medical uses of electricity. Henri François Le Dran and René Jacques Croissant de Garengeot were the authors of standard textbooks of operative surgery.

Among the many interesting cases recorded by Garengeot in his *Treatise of Chirurgical Operations* (1731) is that of the Paris surgeon who successfully replaced a nose that had been bitten off in a fight!

"In the month of September, 1724, a soldier, of the regiment of Conti, coming out of the Epée Royale, from an inn in the corner of the street Deux-Ecus, was attacked by one of his comrades, and, in the struggle had his nose bitten off, so as to remove almost all the cartilaginous part. His adversary, perceiving that he had a bit of flesh in his mouth, spat it out into the gutter, and endeavoured to crush it by trampling upon it. The soldier who, on his part, was not less eager, took up the end of his nose, and threw it into the shop of Monsieur Galin, a brother-practitioner of mine, while he ran after his adversary. During this time Monsieur Galin examined the nose which had been thrown into his shop, and, as it was covered with dirt, he washed it at the well. The soldier returning to be dressed, Monsieur Galin washed his wound and face, which were covered with blood, with a little warm water and then put the extremity of the nose into this liquor, to heat it a little. Having in this manner cleansed the wound, M. Galin now put the nose into its natural situation, and retained it there by means of an agglutinating plaster and bandage. Next day, the union appeared to have taken place; and, on the fourth day, I myself dressed him, with M. Galin, and saw that the extremity of the nose was perfectly united and cicatrized."

Antonio Scarpa of Pavia made important contributions to the subject of hernia and to the surgery of the eye and the ear. He was also one of the greatest medical artists and drew all the illustrations for his own books. Spain produced a great surgeon in the person of Antonio de Gimbernat, who devised an operation for strangulated femoral hernia and also advanced the surgery of the eye, the vascular system, and the urinary organs.

First of the great British surgeons of the century was William Cheselden (1688–1752), surgeon to St. Thomas's Hospital, who won an international reputation as an operator for stone in the bladder. This malady was exceedingly common in former times, it is believed because of the poor and monotonous diet of many sections of the populace. The operation of lithotomy was a very severe one and sufferers from the stone only submitted to it when the pain and discomfort of their condition made life almost unbearable. Up to the time of Cheselden the operation usually performed involved the making of a huge incision in the region of the groin, the dilatation of the neck of the bladder with special instruments, and the forcible extraction of the stone with forceps. The whole procedure often took an hour and in the absence of anaesthesia it must have been a ghastly ordeal for all concerned. Cheselden perfected a new technique which enabled him to complete the operation in one minute (his record time was 54 seconds). He reduced the mortality from about fifty per cent to under ten per cent and his results were not bettered until almost the end of the nineteenth century.

Cheselden's own modest account gives us a fascinating glimpse into the mind of the surgeon and provides some indication of the stress and anxiety to which even the most expert operators are exposed:

"What success I had in my private practice I have kept no account of because I had no intention to publish it, that not being sufficiently witnessed. Publicly in St. Thomas' Hospital I have cut two hundred and thirteen; of the first fifty only three died; of the second fifty, three; of the third fifty, eight; and of the last sixty-three, six. Several of these patients had the smallpox during their cure some of which died, but I think not more in proportion than what usually die of that distemper; these are not reckoned among those who died of the operation. The reason why so few died in the first two fifties was that at that time, few very bad cases offered; in the third, the operation being in high request even the most aged and the most miserable cases expected to be saved by it. One of the three that died out of the one hundred and five was very ill with whooping-cough; another bled to death by an artery into the bladder, it being very hot weather at that time. But this accident taught me afterwards, whenever a vessel bled that I could not find, to dilate the wound with a knife till I could see it.

"If I have any reputation in this way I have earned it dearly, for no one ever endured more anxiety and sickness before an operation, yet from the time I began to operate all uneasiness ceased and if I have had better success than some others I do not impute it to more knowledge but to the happiness of mind that was never ruffled or disconcerted and a hand that never trembled during any operation."

News of Cheselden's remarkable skill and results spread all over Europe. A young French surgeon named Morand was sent over to England in 1729 by the Royal Academy of France to report upon the operation. He states that he often saw a stone removed in twenty-four seconds and that it rarely took more than a minute. He watched Cheselden cut twenty-seven patients without losing one, and spoke so favourably of the method that it soon became known and practised throughout Europe. It remained in ordinary use until 1885, when lithotrity—crushing the stone—came into vogue.

Cheselden was also a great eye surgeon, and on one occasion he restored the sight of a blind boy by constructing an artificial pupil. Independently of the French surgeon Petit, he discovered the method of circular amputation by two incisions. He was a man of extraordinary versatility, and not only drew the illustrations for his own books but designed the original Fulham Bridge which was built across the Thames in 1729. Among his patients were Sir Isaac Newton and Alexander Pope. The latter refers to his surgeon in the lines:

> "I'll do what Mead and Cheselden advise,
> To keep these limbs and to preserve these eyes."

Contemporary with Cheselden was Percivall Pott (1714–1788), surgeon to St. Bartholomew's Hospital for a period of fifty years. Pott's father died when the boy was three years old but thanks to the help of a wealthy relative he was apprenticed when fifteen years of age to Edward Nourse, then assistant surgeon to St. Bartholomew's Hospital. A fee of two hundred guineas was paid in accordance with the custom prevailing at that time. Pott was an apt pupil and in 1736 he obtained the Grand Diploma of the Barber-Surgeons' Company. He was appointed to the staff of St. Bartholomew's Hospital in 1744 and acquired a great reputation as an operator and as a teacher.

In 1758 while riding in Kent Street, Southwark, now the Old Kent Road, Pott was thrown from his horse and sustained a compound fracture of the tibia. The incident was thus described by his son-in-law: "Conscious of the dangers attendant on fractures of this nature and thoroughly aware how much they may be increased by rough treatment or improper position, he would not suffer himself to be moved until he had made the necessary disposition. He sent to Westminster for two chairmen to bring their poles: he patiently lay on the cold pavement, it being the middle of January, until they arrived. In this situation he purchased a door to which he made them nail their poles. When all was ready, he caused himself to be laid on it, and on it was carried home." The distinguished patient was examined by many of his fellow-surgeons, who consulted and concurred that the only course was amputation. However, while the instruments were being got ready Edward Nourse, Pott's old teacher, arrived, and on examining the limb decided that it might be possible to save it. The other surgeons deferred to Nourse's opinion, and Pott retained his leg. In due course the wound healed satisfactorily.

Pott thus had a personal interest in the subject of fractures and it is with a variety of fracture-dislocation of the ankle (Pott's fracture) that his name is always connected. Two other conditions are named after him: Pott's puffy tumour, a condition associated with osteomyelitis of the skull, and Pott's disease, or spinal caries due to tuberculosis. Pott was also the first to describe chimney sweep's cancer—cancer of the scrotum. Pott's lectures made his name known all over Europe. He and Cheselden did much to place surgery on a rational basis and to bring it into line with the new look in physiology and medicine.

An even greater surgeon—indeed one of the leading figures in the whole history of medicine—was John Hunter (1728–1793), the founder of experimental surgery and of surgical pathology. As a young lad Hunter set out on horseback from his home at Long Calderwood near Glasgow to join his elder brother William, who had already established himself as a teacher of anatomy and midwifery in London. After studying under Cheselden and Pott he spent four years as an army surgeon. When he did settle down in London he taught in his brother's school and commenced his researches in comparative anatomy and physiology. After a time he was able to set up a large establishment in Leicester Square on the site of the present Odeon cinema, which comprised his home, his consulting rooms, museum and lecture theatre. He also had a country home at Earl's Court where he kept an extensive collection of birds and beasts which he studied in life and dissected after death. His animals included lions, tigers and giraffes and a bison, with which he used to wrestle. He got up at four in the morning to dissect and his observations ranged from insects to whales. The great museum which he formed eventually contained more than thirteen thousand specimens. It was purchased for the nation and deposited in the Royal College of Surgeons where the greater part of it, rehabilitated after wartime bombing, may still be seen. Among the objects of interest in the Hunterian museum is the Skeleton of Byrne, the Irish giant, which Hunter long coveted and at last secured for five hundred pounds after the owner's death. John Hunter ranks as the founder of modern surgery because of the vast range of his observations and because of the enormous influence which he exerted on his pupils. These latter included such great men as Edward Jenner, the discoverer of vaccination, John Abernethy and Sir Astley Cooper. Hunter elevated surgery to the rank of a science through his intensive study of anatomy and of changes in function and structure of disease. He made an exhaustive study of the nature of inflammation and he was the founder of experimental surgery.

John Hunter was so passionately devoted to observation and research that he often grudged the time which he had to spend seeing patients or operating. But although he often expressed his distaste for "chasing that damned guinea" he always responded to a call and was a first-rate operator. He explored the treatment of club-foot and of ruptured tendons after having ruptured his own Achilles tendon. Having experimented on the circulation of the blood in stags' antlers in the Royal Park at Windsor, he devised an operation for treating aneurysms with a ligature instead of by amputation. He was for many years surgeon to St. George's Hospital, and it was in the board room of the hospital that he died suddenly in 1793.

Samuel Sharp, a pupil of Cheselden, was a famous surgeon to Guy's Hospital. He was the first to cut the cornea with a knife in operating for cataract.

British surgery was not connected with any one centre and some of the greatest improvements were made by provincial practitioners. Charles White of Manchester and Henry Park of Liverpool were very notable practitioners of conservative surgery towards the end of the eighteenth century. Almost simultaneously they introduced a new operation for excising diseased bones and joints and thus obviated amputation.

Alexander Monro (1697–1767), son of John Monro, an army surgeon, is regarded as the father of the Edinburgh Medical School. He taught surgery and anatomy for thirty-eight years and conducted a large practice. On one occasion he was in-

THE EIGHTEENTH CENTURY 123

volved in a public demonstration against "body snatching", following a fight between his students and the relatives of a woman who had just been hanged. While the fight was in progress, the "body" came to life, and lived for many years, being known as "Half-hangit Maggie Dickson". Alexander Monro was succeeded by his son, Alexander Monro the second, who achieved even greater fame than his father; and in due course the professorship passed to the grandson, Alexander Monro the third.

Benjamin Bell (1749–1806) had been described as the first of the Edinburgh scientific surgeons. He wrote a great text-book of surgery in six volumes, which was translated into French and German.

Appendicectomy is now the commonest of all abdominal operations, yet the history of the surgery of the appendix does not go back much more than two hundred years and operation as a routine measure has only been undertaken during the present century. The term "appendicitis" was coined by Reginald Heber Fitz, a Boston surgeon, in 1886. Long before this date we can find descriptions of the appendix as an anatomical organ and discussions as to its function. There are also a number of early reports of what may or may not have been cases of appendicitis. The disease has probably always been common although its exact nature and importance were not realized. It is very probable that many of the cases described by the older writers on medicine as the "iliac passion" and the "cholic passion" were in fact cases of appendicitis, but the terms were used with reference to almost any kind of pain in the right lower abdomen. It is quite possible that appendix abscesses were occasionally evacuated. The doubtful nature of most of the early case reports is shown by a report of Aretaeus, a Greek physician of the second century A.D.: "I once made an opening into an abscess in the colon on the right side near the liver, and much pus rushed out, and much also by the kidneys and bladder for several days, and the man recovered."

An important landmark in the history of appendicitis is the publication of the earliest post-mortem report, by Lorenz Heister, a famous German surgeon, in 1718. Heister recorded that in November 1711 when he was dissecting the body of a malefactor in the public anatomical theatre at Altdorf, "I found the small guts very red and inflamed in several places, insomuch that the smallest vessels were as beautifully filled with blood as if they had been injected with red wax . . . but, when I was about to demonstrate the situation of the great guts, I found the vermiform process of the caecum preternaturally black, adhering closer to the peritoneum than usual. As I now was about to separate it, by gently pulling it asunder, the membranes of this process broke, notwithstanding the body was quite fresh, and discharged two or three spoonfulls of matter. This instance may stand as a proof of the possibility of inflammation arising, and abscesses forming, in the appendicular, as well as in other parts of the body, which I have not observed to be much noticed by other writers; and when, in practice, we meet with a burning and pain where this part is situated, we ought to give attention to it."

The honour of being the first to record a successful appendicectomy belongs to a British surgeon, Claudius Amyand, sergeant-surgeon to George II. Amyand's case was reported to the Royal Society and published in its Transactions in 1736 under the title: "Of an Inguinal Rupture, with a Pin in the Appendix Caeci, encrusted with Stone, and some Observations on Wounds in the Guts." The patient was a boy of eleven, named Hanvil Anderson, and the hernia had been present from infancy. Amyand decided that an associated faecal fistula could be cured only by cure of the hernia. On 6 December, 1735, he explored the scrotal swelling and found the appendix perforated by an encrusted pin. The appendix, which was doubled on itself, was amputated and a stump one inch long was left because a fistula was anticipated. The hernial sac was removed and the fistulous tract excised. Healing was rapid and the stump ligature separated on the tenth day without incident. "Tis easy to conceive," wrote Amyand, "that this operation was as painful to the patient as laborious to me: it was a continued dissection, attended with danger on parts not well distinguished: it lasted near half an hour, and the patient bore it with great courage."

One or two further reports on disease of the appendix

appeared in the eighteenth century, and they became fairly common after about 1830 (see page 144).

Claudius Amyand was the second son of Isaac Amyand, a Huguenot refugee who was naturalized in London in 1688. Claudius himself was naturalized in 1700. As an apprentice surgeon he went to the wars in Flanders and in 1704 took part in the battle of Blenheim receiving £30 as his share of the bounty. In addition to holding the office of serjeant-surgeon to George II, he was principal surgeon to St. George's Hospital and to the Westminster Hospital, and Master of the Barber-Surgeons' Company. Amyand was one of the pioneers of inoculation for smallpox in this country. In 1722 Princess Caroline, wife of the future George II, wanted to protect her children against smallpox by means of inoculation, the practice of which had been introduced into England in 1721 by her friend, Lady Mary Wortley Montagu. She persuaded George I to allow experimental inoculations on six condemned felons, on condition that they should be pardoned afterwards. Five of the criminals contracted the disease in mild form and recovered, the sixth concealed the fact that he had previously had smallpox and so was not infected. All six escaped the hangman. The Princess then had eleven children from the charity ward of the parish of St. James inoculated by Amyand and this too proved successful. On 17 April, 1722, the Princesses Caroline, aged nine, and Amelia, aged eleven, were inoculated by Amyand, under the watchful eye of the Royal Physician, Sir Hans Sloane—fortunately with success.

Smallpox was at this time a terrible disease which killed one in four of those attacked and disfigured the majority of those who survived. In the graphic words of Macaulay: "The smallpox was always present, filling the churchyard with corpses, tormenting with constant fears all whom it had not yet stricken, leaving on those whose lives it spared the hideous traces of its path; turning the babe into a changeling at which the mother shuddered, and making the eyes and cheeks of the betrothed maiden objects of horror to the lover."

Once the success of inoculation in preventing, or at least greatly mitigating, the power of this loathsome disease had been established there was naturally a tremendous demand

for the operation. Claudius Amyand was one of the first
English surgeons to inoculate on a large scale, but his fame in
this respect was surpassed by that of Daniel Sutton of Ingate-
stone and Thomas Dimsdale of Hertford. Dimsdale, who was
in 1768 summoned to Russia to inoculate the Empress Catherine
the Great and her son, received a fee of £10,000, a pension of
£500, and a Barony. The object of inoculation was to give the
patient a mild attack of smallpox which would confer immunity
against any further attacks. The practice was not without
danger and after 1798 it gave place to Jenner's method of
vaccination, whereby the patient was rendered immune not
by being infected with true smallpox but with a milder form
of the disease, known as cowpox or vaccinia.

Reference has already been made to Lorenz Heister's
account of appendicitis. The writings of this great surgeon, who
was professor of surgery and anatomy at Altdorf in Germany,
provide us with many fascinating glimpses of eighteenth-
century practice. Heister published in 1718 a *Surgery* which is
one of the earliest systematic treatises on the subject and is
especially interesting for its illustrations. This work was so
valuable as a textbook that it passed through innumerable
editions and was translated into almost every European language. Later in life, Heister published a large volume of *Medical,
Chirurgical and Anatomical Cases and Observations*, an English
translation of which appeared in 1755. This book contains
a good deal of autobiographical matter, especially concerning
Heister's younger days when he sought experience as an
army surgeon and also visited hospitals and medical schools in
Holland, France, and England. So keen was he on seeing operations that he frequented the great fairs to which itinerant
operators resorted in large numbers. Some of these wandering
surgeons undertook operations which the more regular practitioners of the time did not dare to perform, and Heister was
not too proud to learn from them. In the year 1700, when he
was a lad of seventeen, Heister visited the fair at Frankfort
and this is his description of what he saw:

"It is usual for a number of oculists, and other operators,
to resort to Frankfort at the fair time, to undertake the

cure of persons afflicted with ruptures, cataracts, the stone, excrescences, hare-lips, and such like disorders; there being, at the time I am speaking of, no physician or surgeon at Frankfort who cared to perform these operations. One Eisenbart, at that time very famous, came among the rest. As I soon saw the necessity and use of attending such operations, I embraced every opportunity of being present, that I might learn and improve as much as possible by what I then observed. In the year 1700, at the Easter Fair, a boy about nine years of age, afflicted with a rupture, was brought by his parents to one of these empirics, as they could meet with no other assistance in Frankfort, begging of him to perform the operation on their child. These sort of people do not attempt the cure of their patients with trusses, because they seldom remain longer than the fair lasts, and in that short time, there is no possibility of effecting the cure with a truss; besides, if it had been in their power, it was what they did not choose on another account, the pay for a cure by a truss not exceeding ten shillings at most, whereas the operation was rated higher, and amounted to five or ten pounds or more, according to the patient's circumstances, they therefore, as it was their livelihood, always recommended the operation. This itinerant physician accordingly undertook his cure, and, after previous purging, performed the operation the next day in the following manner."

Heister then describes how the operator pushed the prolapsed intestine back into the abdomen, opened the scrotum, and ligated and removed the testicle. The wound was filled with lint and a vulnerary plaster, compress and bandage were applied. A proper diet was recommended. The child made rapid progress and there were no complications. In about three weeks the wound was perfectly healed.

Heister saw this same Eisenbart perform a more formidable operation for the removal of a tumour from the face:

"A sturdy fat woman, a farmer's wife, about thirty years of age, had a large frightful moveable tumour on her left cheek, extending itself to the ear and chin, which became very troublesome, and daily increasing in bulk, and as nobody else would undertake to discuss or extirpate it, she applied to the before-mentioned empiric, to know if he could effect a cure. He accordingly took her under his care, and having purged her previous to the operation, he placed her on a chair, the assistants keeping her fast, and made a longitudinal incision through the skin from the top to the bottom, and then made another smaller directly across the middle of the first, separating the flaps, sometimes with his knife, and sometimes with his finger, to the base; then passing a crooked needle and thread through the tumour, with which pulling it towards him, he disengaged it by degrees on all sides where it adhered, frequently wiping up the blood with a sponge, and compressing with his finger those veins which bled too freely, till he had entirely dissected the tumour away; two arteries bleeding, he applied to their orifices a little piece of vitriol wrapped up in a linen rag, and filled up the wound with lint and sponge, over which he laid three large linen compresses, applying a double-headed bandage three fingers breadth about her head, and ordered her to go to bed."

The patient was not dressed till the fourth day and the cure was happily effected, but not, we are told, without a great scar.

Heister several times witnessed the operation of couching or depressing cataract, and he says that the itinerant operators had little success despite their claims. He saw the Chevalier Taylor, the most notorious of all the itinerant oculists, many times, and states that of the hundreds he couched in the years 1750–52 in the principal cities of Germany, not one in a hundred recovered their sight. The operation was often performed when the cataract was not "ripe", that is to say not hard enough and not therefore amenable to surgery.

At Amsterdam Heister saw his first operation for harelip performed on a child of two by Mr. Van Bortel, an eminent surgeon of the city, whose procedure was as follows:

"He ordered one of his assistants to seat himself on a chair, and take the child on his lap, holding it fast round the waist, at the same time confining the child's hands. Another assistant stood behind, holding his head on both sides to keep it steady. A third held the child's right leg, and a fourth the left, whereby he was fixed immoveable. Then taking a good pair of scissors in his right hand, and with the index-finger and thumb of the left, taking hold of one edge of the fissure, he cut off about as much as the breadth of the back of a knife, and the same he immediately did on the other edge; then wiping off the blood from the mouth and lip with a sponge, and having three proper needles ready, he passed the first through both lips of the fissure, about the breadth of the back of the knife from the edge of the wound, the second in the middle, and the third at the bottom, and fixing a double thread to the uppermost, he twisted it backwards and forwards several times, and in the same manner to the two other needles; after rubbing the wound with a little honey of roses, he applied a narrow bandage from the part to the back of the head, bringing it round to the forehead, where he tied it, and pinned it fast to the child's cap behind, and on each side. The fifth day the middle needle was removed; the sixth day the uppermost, and on the seventh the other; after anointing the part with vulnerary balsam, he applied a narrow strip of plaster to the part, upon the falling off of which, the wound was perfectly healed."

Heister, like nearly all great surgeons, used few and simple instruments. "In every operation of surgery," he said, "that method which is performed with the fewest and most simple instruments is to be preferred to a great apparatus difficult to be applied, as most of these have been invented more for the sake of pomp than real utility." He makes exceptions in the case of the instruments required for such special operations as lithotomy and trepanation and himself advocated the use of a special concealed lancet for taking out tonsils.

"I know well," he wrote, "that suppurated tonsils may be opened with a lancet or sharp knife; yet for the sake of children and the more delicate and timorous, particular of the fair sex, we ought to contrive a milder method, as these frequently and obstinately oppose cutting or puncturing with instruments, to be suffocated than suffer themselves to be touched. In which case I think it in nowise repugnant to the wisdom, duty, and conscience of a physician to use deceit in order to save the life of his patient, and to free him quickly from his pain. For a physician must do everything which can in any wise contribute towards preserving the life of his patient. An instrument maker at Amsterdam showed me a new instrument for opening suppurated tonsils, the inventor of which is unknown to me, with which we may practise an honest deceit upon such a patient. For after the surgeon has introduced into the mouth this instrument (which appears like a spatula and in which is contained the lancet) to depress the tongue to look at the throat, he may push forward the lancet with the thumb, and open the tumour and the patient hardly know anything of the matter."

FOR FURTHER READING

Comrie, J. D. *History of Scottish Medicine*. 2 vols. 1932.

Cope, Sir Z. *William Cheselden, 1688–1752*. Edinburgh. 1953.

Creese, P. G. The first appendicectomy. *Surg. Gynec. Obstet.*, 1953, *97*, 643.

Laignel-Lavastine, M. and Molinery, R. *French Medicine* (Clio Medica). New York. 1934.

Lloyd, G. M. The life and works of Percivall Pott. *St. Barth. Hosp. Rep.*, 1933, *66*, 291.

Paget, S. *John Hunter, Man of Science and Surgeon*. 1897.

Peachey, G. C. *A Memoir of William and John Hunter*. 1924.

Shepherd, J. A. Acute appendicitis: a historical survey. *Lancet*, 1954, ii, 299.

Thomson, S. C. The Great Windmill Street School. *Bull. Hist. Med.*, 1942, *12*, 377.

Wall, C. *History of the Surgeons' Company, 1745–1800*. 1937.

CHAPTER EIGHT

Early Nineteenth Century

EARLY nineteenth-century surgery was mainly a continuation of the surgery of the eighteenth century, but the centre of advance shifted from Paris to London. The great John Hunter had died in 1793 but his influence was still paramount. Nearly all the leading British surgeons of the period had been his pupils, and this meant that they had received a thorough training in anatomy and physiology and in the new science of surgical pathology, which Hunter had created. There was a much better understanding of the actual processes of disease, and symptoms and signs observed during the course of illness were beginning to be correlated with changes revealed at post-mortem examination. Improvements were made in methods of examination of patients and in record-keeping. As always, medicine and surgery derived great benefit from contemporary advances in pure science, especially of course from chemistry and physics. These changes did not all come at once and there were no revolutionary developments in the early years of the century, but medicine gradually began to take on a more scientific character. In some directions progress was very slow. Thus, although the stethoscope was introduced in 1819, the modern clinical thermometer was not made until 1867. Blood transfusion, the potential value of which had been demonstrated in the seventeenth century, was revived in 1818 but was not carried out on any scale until the time of the American Civil War. Surgical anaesthesia by means of ether and chloroform did not come until 1846 and 1847 respectively, and antisepsis not until after the turn of the century. In the absence of anaes-thesia and antisepsis there was no general operating within the head, the abdomen, or the female pelvis, although records of a few such interventions bear witness to the courage and for-titude of patient and surgeon alike. War continued to be the great school for the surgeon. The long-drawn-out Napoleonic campaigns provided endless scope for the observation and treatment of every type of injury. Many bold operative feats were performed by the surgeons on both sides, especially in the treatment of gunshot wounds.

Interscapulo-thoracic amputation (total removal of the arm, shoulder-blade and collar-bone) was performed for the first time by Ralph Cuming, a surgeon in the Royal Navy, in 1808. The patient was a young sailor of twenty-one who had been hit by a cannon ball, and the operation was carried out in the naval hospital at Antigua in the West Indies. The conditions under which the operation was performed were primitive and everything was rendered more difficult by the terrible heat. There is no mention of any form of anaesthesia or of any anti-septic precautions. The boiling of instruments after contact with septic cases had been advised but was not always carried out; knives were sometimes scalded because it was believed that warm instruments inflicted less pain than cold steel. Opium or rum was sometimes used for analgesia but this was exceptional, and there is no mention of it in this case. It was customary to administer laudanum to the patient after operation and wine was often given every two or three hours in the postoperative period. In operating Cuming had to subordinate everything to speed, not only because of the necessity for minimizing pain and shock but also because of the haemorrhage that would occur from so large an area. As one of his contemporaries put it, "The knife is to be handled more like a sabre than a surgeon's scalpel." Haemostatic forceps had not been invented and Cuming had to grasp the great vessels between finger and thumb while his assistant placed a ligature around them. Silk had recently displaced waxed thread for this purpose. When the wound was finally closed, the edges were held in accurate contact with adhesive straps, and a dressing in the form of a poultice was applied. The poultice would be held in place by long strips of adhesive plaster reaching across the back and chest, and covered by a spica bandage. Cuming's patient made a complete recovery and after being invalided to England he was shown to the students of St. Bartholomew's Hospital.

It is hard to realize what a major surgical operation must have meant to the patient in the days before anaesthesia, and special interest therefore attaches to a personal account of an operation for the removal of a stone from the bladder. The operation was performed by Henry Cline, surgeon to St. Thomas's Hospital and one of the leading operators of the day, on 30 December, 1811. The anonymous patient thus describes his ordeal:

"My habit and constitution being good it required little preparation of body, and my mind was made up. When all parties had arrived I retired to my room for a minute, bent my knee in silent adoration and submission and returning to the surgeons conducted them to the apartment in which the preparations had been made. The bandages &c. having been adjusted I was prepared to receive a shock of pain of extreme violence and so much had I over-rated it, that the first incision did not even make me wince although I had declared that it was not my intention to restrain such impulse, convinced that such effort of restraint could only lead to additional exhaustion. At subsequent moments, therefore I did cry out under the pain, but was allowed to have gone through the operation with great firmness.

"The forcing up of the staff prior to the introduction of the gorget gave me the first real pain, but this instantly subsided after the incision of the bladder was made, the rush of urine appeared to relieve it and soothe the wound.

"When the forceps was introduced the pain was again very considerable and every movement of the instrument in endeavouring to find the stone increased it. Still, however, my mind was firm and confident, and, although anxious, I was yet alive to what was going on. After several ineffectual attempts to grasp the stone I heard the operator say in the lowest whisper, 'It is a little awkward, it lies under my hand. Give me the curved forceps', upon which he withdrew the others. Here, I think, I asked if there was anything wrong— or something to that purport—and was reanimated by the reply conveyed in the kindest manner, 'Be patient, Sir, it will soon be over'. When the other forceps was introduced I had again to undergo the searching for the stone and heard Mr. Cline say, 'I have got it'. I had probably by this time conceived that the worst was over; but when the necessary force was applied to withdraw the stone the sensation was such as I cannot find words to describe. In addition to the positive pain there was something peculiar in the feel. The bladder embraced the stone as firmly as the stone was itself grasped by the forceps; it seemed as if the whole organ was about to be torn out. The duration, however, of this really trying part of the operation was short and when the words 'Now, Sir, it is all over' struck my ear, the ejaculation of 'Thank God! Thank God!' was uttered with a fervency and fulness of heart which can only be conceived. I am quite unable to describe my sensations at the moment. There was a feeling of release, not from the pain of the operation, for that was gone and lost sight of, but from my enemy and tormentor with a lightness and buoyancy of spirits, elating my imagination to the belief that I was restored to perfect health as if by a miracle.

"I never heard what was the precise duration of the operation but conceive it to have been between twelve and fifteen minutes. With respect to the pain I am persuaded that if it were possible to concentrate what I have often suffered in one night into the same space of time it would have been less endurable. Indeed, this difference between the operation and one night's endurance of the stone was manifest. I have often been most distressingly reduced by the latter, but was not exhausted in the slightest degree by the former; at least my mind was firm throughout, and my body was not sensibly enfeebled. Upon the whole should I be again similarly afflicted, I should not hesitate in again submitting myself to the same mode of relief provided I could place myself in equally capable hands."

It is pleasant to know that this plucky patient had sufficiently recovered by the end of a month to be able to walk nearly two miles and that he was perfectly cured at the end of the sixth week from the day of the operation.

Interest in plastic surgery, which had made little advance since the sixteenth century, was revived by reports coming from India, the original home of the specialty. The *Gentleman's*

Magazine of October 1794 contained an illustrated account of a rhinoplastic operation upon one Cowasjee, a bullock-driver. This man had served as a driver with the English Army in 1792 and had been made prisoner by Tippoo Sahib, who cut off his nose and one of his hands. He subsequently became a pensioner of the East India Company, but remained without a nose for twelve months, when a new one was constructed by a native operator near Poona. About the same time a British surgeon, Mr. Lucas of Madras, performed a similar operation by the ancient Hindu method. News of these successes led Joseph Constantine Carpue, a noted surgeon and teacher of anatomy in London, to perform the first rhinoplastic operations in Europe in modern times. Using the old Hindu method of taking a flap of skin from the forehead he operated successfully upon two patients in October 1814 and January 1815. In 1816 Carpue published *An Account of two Successful Operations for Restoring a Lost Nose*, a work which is regarded as one of the greatest landmarks in the history of reconstructive surgery. After Carpue, modern plastic surgery owes much to Carl Ferdinand von Graefe (1787–1840), professor of surgery at Berlin, who devised the operation for congenital cleft-palate and carried out pioneer work on the surgery of the eyelids. Von Graefe was also the first German surgeon to excise the lower jaw and he improved the technique of Caesarean section.

The leading British surgeons of the pre-Listerian era were John and Charles Bell, Sir Astley Cooper, John Abernethy, Charles Aston Key, Benjamin Travers, Sir Benjamin Brodie, Robert Liston, George James Guthrie, Abraham Colles, and James Syme. These men all practised surgery in a scientific spirit and made outstanding contributions to knowledge.

Most popular of all London surgeons during the first quarter of the century was Sir Astley Paston Cooper (1768–1841), a Norfolk man and a pupil of John Hunter. He was a pioneer in the surgery of blood vessels, in experimental surgery, and in the surgery of the ear. In 1808 he successfully ligated the common carotid and the external iliac arteries for aneurysm, and in 1817 he accomplished his celebrated feat of ligating the abdominal aorta. The latter operation, which was carried out in Guy's Hospital upon a patient who was in imminent danger of bleeding to death from an enormous aneurysm, involved the arrest of the circulation through the main channel of supply to the lower half of the body. The patient survived for only forty hours but Cooper had demonstrated the feasibility of the operation and its probable beneficial effect in a less advanced case of aneurysm. In actual fact the first successful operation of this kind was not reported until just over a century later.

Another of Astley Cooper's great feats was an amputation at the hip joint, carried out at Guy's Hospital on 16 January, 1824, and reported in the *Lancet* as follows:

"This formidable operation was performed here this morning, for the first time, by Sir Astley Cooper, in the presence of some of the surgeons and pupils belonging to these institutions. The number of those present, however, was not so great as on many other occasions; no previous notice of the operation having been given, owing to its having been determined on but a few minutes before it was performed. The patient is a man about 40 years of age, whose leg had been amputated some few years ago, just above the knee: since which time the thigh-bone has become diseased from the extremity of the stump up to the trochanter major, and this disease has had such effect on him of late, that he has been rapidly sinking under it. The thigh was of the middle size. On being asked this morning to submit to an operation, he readily consented. At half past one the patient was brought into the operating theatre, and placed in the recumbent position on the table. The femoral artery was first cut down upon, and secured about one inch and a half below Poupart's ligament, but it was discovered, by passing the finger deep between the triceps and vastus internus, that the profunda was still pulsating and it was evident the profunda was given off higher than usual, which obliged Sir Astley to secure the femoral artery almost close to Poupart's ligament. Sir Astley, standing to the outer side, with the limb in one hand and the catling in the other, commenced the operation by making an incision just below Poupart's ligament, a little to the iliac side of the femoral artery; this was continued obliquely downwards and outwards to the back of the thigh, about one third of the way down, from which point the knife was carried in the opposite direction, obliquely upwards and inwards to meet the first incision; by this means forming an elliptical curve. The cellular membrane was merely cut through at first, but the knife was again carried in the same direction as before, and thus the muscles were also separated; at this step of the operation it was necessary to apply another ligature on the inside of the limb; here the operator changed positions and sat on the chair in front of the patient, and waited a short time to see whether there were any bleeding vessels. After the lapse of a few minutes, the operation was continued, the head of the thigh-bone being removed from the acetabulum without any difficulty. Two ligatures in addition to those already used were applied, making in the whole four; the integuments were brought together, and a suture applied to the upper portion; strips of adhesive plaster, and lastly a bandage were put over the stump: about 12 ounces of blood were lost, but it had the appearance of being venous. The limb was removed in the space of twenty minutes, the securing of the arteries and the dressings occupied fifteen more; the whole was, therefore, completed in thirty-five minutes. During the operation the man was extremely faint; but some wine being given him and some fresh air admitted, he recovered. The patient bore the operation with extraordinary fortitude; and after all was finished, he said to Sir Astley, 'that it was the hardest day's work he had ever gone through', to which Sir Astley replied, 'that it was almost the hardest he ever had.' "

Astley Cooper's books on hernia, on injuries of the joints, on diseases of the testis, and on the thymus gland are surgical classics. Although the modern use of sterilized catgut was introduced by Lister in 1868, Astley Cooper had used this substance in 1817.

Sir Astley's daily routine was to rise at six and to work in his private dissecting room until eight. He himself wrote: "If I laid my head upon my pillow at night, without having dissected something in the day, I should think that I had lost that day." This passion for dissecting Cooper shared with all his colleagues, especially those who had, like himself, been pupils of John Hunter. After breakfasting on two hot buttered rolls and tea, he saw poor patients until nine, and then attended to his own consulting practice until one. His carriage would then take him rapidly to Guy's Hospital for ward visits. At two he lectured on anatomy at nearby St. Thomas's Hospital, after which he went through the dissecting rooms with the students or operated. Visits or operations on private patients occupied him until seven, when he had his dinner and perhaps took a nap for a few minutes. A further round of visits very often kept him busy until midnight.

Sir Astley Cooper was an excellent diagnostician and he possessed to an exceptional degree that power of inspiring confidence which is the hallmark of the truly great physician or surgeon. He was certainly a bold and rapid operator, but according to his own estimate was not good at operations requiring delicacy. His colleagues were in no doubt about his supreme skill and the students idolized him. Fortunately, we have a contemporary description of the impact made by the great surgeon upon those who awaited his coming in the operating theatre at Guy's Hospital:

"Profound silence obtained upon his entry, that person so manly and so truly imposing, and the awful feeling connected with the occasion can never be forgotten by any of his pupils. The elegance of his operation, without the slightest affectation, all ease, all kindness to the patients, and equally solicitous that nothing should be hidden from the observation of the pupils, rapid in execution, masterly in manner, no hurry, no disorder, the most trifling minutiae attended to, the dressing generally applied by his own hand, the light and elegant manner in which Sir Astley Cooper employed his instruments, always astonished me."

In 1820 Cooper was called to see King George IV, who was suffering from a small tumour—a sebaceous cyst—on his scalp. The cyst was tender and inflamed and it was growing larger, but the surgeons advised delay. Even the most trifling operation becomes a matter for serious consideration when the patient is a monarch—and patients had been known to die of erysipelas after the removal of tumours of this type. The King was all for action and one day when Astley Cooper had been summoned to Brighton his sovereign came into his bedroom at one o'clock in the morning saying, "I am now ready to have it done. I wish you to remove this thing from my head." To which the surgeon replied, "Sire—not for the world now—your life is too important to have so serious a thing done in a corner." George was not to be put off indefinitely and a little later a day was fixed for the operation to be performed at Windsor. Two of the royal physicians and four surgeons were present, but there was still a delicate point of professional etiquette to be settled. According to all the rules, the operation should have been performed by the Serjeant-Surgeon, Sir Everard Home, but he declined the honour, as did the surgeon next in seniority, Henry Cline, who had been one of Astley Cooper's teachers. The King, however, insisted that Cooper should do the operation and demanded:' 'Where am I to sit?'

The rest of the story is told by Sir Astley Cooper: "Here, Sire, taking a chair to the window, and begging an instrument of Home, I made an incision in the scalp, and upon the side on which I stood, which was about three-fourths of its size, I with difficulty detached it from the skin without cutting the skin itself. On that side on which Cline stood I begged him to detach it, which he did, but it took up a great deal of time on the whole. The edges of the wound were brought together, and lint and plaister applied. The King bore the operation well, requested that there might be no hurry, and when it was finished, said, 'What do you call the tumour?' I said, 'A *steatome*, Sire.' 'Then,' said he, 'I hope it will *stay at home*, and not annoy me any more.' "

The operation was performed on a Wednesday and all went well until Saturday, when the King complained: "I have not slept all night, and I am damned bad this morning; my head is sore all over." The next day he had a severe attack of gout but his head was no longer sore and it soon healed. For this service Astley Cooper was made a Baronet and the King gave him a beautiful epergne which cost him 500 guineas.

Cooper attributed his professional success to his uniform and unfailing courtesy to rich and poor alike, as well as to his zeal and industry. In one year his income was £21,000. His largest fee, a thousand guineas, was tossed to him by Mr. Hyatt, a rich West Indian planter, in his nightcap, after a successful operation for stone.

The progress of medicine and surgery was greatly handicapped at this time by the lack of bodies for dissection. As there was no regular and legal source of supply, except a few bodies of executed criminals, the needs of the medical schools were met by "Resurrectionists" or "Body Snatchers" who sold the bodies which they "resurrected" from newly made graves. Sir Astley Cooper was a great patron of the resurrection men and he once stated in evidence before a House of Commons committee that "There is no person, let his situation in life be what it may, whom, if I were disposed to dissect, I could not obtain." The increasing scandal of the black market in human corpses led to a great public outcry, and when Burke and Hare and others resorted to murder in order to keep up the supply of subjects Parliament was at last goaded into action. The Anatomy Act of 1832 went far to remedy the evil and it put the resurrectionists out of business.

Prominent among the surgeons of the early part of the nineteenth century were the brothers John and Charles Bell of Edinburgh and London. John Bell (1763–1820) was one of the founders of surgical anatomy. As a young Fellow of the College of Surgeons of Edinburgh he became very critical of the way in which anatomy was taught by means of formal lectures and he gave voice to his dissatisfaction in his *Letters on the Education of a Surgeon*, published in 1810: "In Dr. Monro's class, unless there be a fortunate succession of bloody murders, not three subjects are dissected in the year. On the remains of a subject fished up from the bottom of a tub of spirits, are demonstrated those delicate nerves which are to be avoided or divided in our operations, and these are demonstrated at the distance of 100 feet! Nerves and arteries which the surgeon has to dissect at the peril of his patient's life."

John Bell therefore began to teach and in 1790 he built his own anatomical school. He was, like his younger brother Charles, a talented artist and was able to illustrate his demonstrations and lectures by his own drawings. For the first time anatomy was taught not only from the purely structural point of view but also with reference to the practical needs of the operating surgeon. Students flocked to Bell's classes, but his very success was his undoing in that it brought upon him the jealousy and enmity of almost the whole medical faculty of Edinburgh. Professional quarrels were then carried on in a manner which would be unthinkable at the present day. Bills were stuck up warning the students against attending Bell's lectures, and his bitterest opponent, Dr. James Gregory, the professor of medicine, wrote: "Any man, if himself or his family were sick, should as soon think of calling in a mad dog as Mr. John Bell." Gregory's party was sufficiently powerful to prevent Bell from obtaining a place on the staff of the Royal Infirmary and he was forced to give up his teaching. He therefore confined himself to surgical practice, in which he achieved success far exceeding that of any of his rivals. John Bell's *Anatomy of the Human Body* and his *Engravings*, illustrating the different parts and organs of the body, contained his own drawings and etchings. In the field of practical surgery he wrote *Discourses on the Nature and Cure of Wounds* (1795) and *Principles of Surgery* (1801–7), the latter work being embellished by his own very fine engravings. Towards the end of his life, John Bell went to Italy and his posthumously published *Observations on Italy* (1825) is one of the best of the many fine travel books written by medical men.

Sir Charles Bell (1774–1842) occupies an even higher place in medical history than his brother. He was, like John, a very talented artist and while still a student at Edinburgh he published a *System of Dissections* illustrated by his own drawings. At the age of thirty he decided to try his fortune in London but he had a hard struggle to establish himself there. His book *On the Anatomy of Expression* (1806), a work intended for artists, established his reputation and he was able to acquire a large house in Leicester Square where he lived and practised. In 1812 he became the sole proprietor of the famous Great Windmill Street School of Anatomy which had been founded by William Hunter.

The fame of Sir Charles Bell rests mainly upon his discovery that definite nerves have a definite course from some part of the brain to a certain peripheral part and, further, that there are two quite distinct kinds of nerves, sensory and motor. This discovery has been described as the greatest made in physiology next to Harvey's demonstration of the circulation of the blood. Sir Charles Bell was also responsible for the original description of the distressing condition known as "Bell's palsy"—facial paralysis due to involvement of the seventh cranial nerve. In 1812 Bell achieved his great ambition of being appointed to the surgical staff of the Middlesex Hospital. He added to the already high reputation of the Hospital and founded its Medical School. After the battle of Waterloo (18 June, 1815) Bell went to Brussels and was placed in charge of a hospital. He operated for three successive days and nights, with only a few brief periods of rest, until his "clothes were stiff with blood and his arms powerless with the exertion of using the knife." When the emergency was over he made a wonderful series of water-colour drawings of the different kinds of wounds and injuries which had come under his observation. These drawings are still preserved in the museum of the Royal Army Medical College in London.

John Abernethy (1764–1831), a pupil of John Hunter, succeeded to the great part of his teacher's practice and won fame and fortune in the early years of the century. Innumerable stories are told of his brusque manner, but, like Dr. Samuel Johnson, he "had nothing of the bear but his skin". "Live on sixpence a day, and earn it" was his advice, and excellent advice it was for many of his pampered patients. Abernethy thought that many diseases were due to digestive disturbances and he treated nearly everything by calomel and blue pill. He was nevertheless a bold and skilful surgeon, and he was, in 1796, the first to ligate the external iliac artery for aneurysm.

Charles Aston Key (1793–1849) was one of Astley Cooper's junior colleagues at Guy's Hospital. He was a swift, neat operator and a popular teacher, and he made improvements in the operations for stone in the bladder and hernia. Benjamin

Travers (1783–1858), another pupil of Sir Astley Cooper, was one of the first hospital surgeons to take a special interest in ophthalmology. In 1820 he published a book on diseases of the eye which was for many years the best systematic treatise on the subject in English.

Robert Liston (1794–1847), surgeon to University College Hospital, was one of the most brilliant and skilful operators of his time. He was especially noted for his rapidity and his students were in the habit of timing his operations with a stop-watch. A tall and powerfully-built man, he was possessed of such strength that he could amputate the thigh with the aid of one assistant, compressing the artery with his left hand and doing all the cutting and sawing with his right. Liston introduced new methods of amputation and invented a special shoe for club-foot. His long splint was the standard treatment of fractures for nearly a hundred years. One of his greatest claims to fame is that he was, in December 1846, the first surgeon in Europe to perform a major surgical operation under anaesthesia (see page 161).

Abraham Colles (1773–1843), Professor of Surgery in Dublin, was the leading Irish surgeon of his day. He was a masterly operator and an inspiring teacher. His treatises on surgical anatomy and on surgery were valued works, but he is mainly remembered for his description of fracture of the lower end of the radius—now universally known as a "Colles fracture".

Sir Benjamin Collins Brodie (1783–1862), a pupil of Sir Everard Home, lectured in the Great Windmill School of Anatomy and later became surgeon to St. George's Hospital. He was a great conservative surgeon, who considered that "his vocation was more to heal limbs than to remove them". The acknowledged leader of the surgical profession in London, his annual income for many years exceeded £10,000—an enormous sum when the value of money in his day is considered. Brodie was a tireless surgeon, research worker, and teacher, and a man of high ideals. He enjoyed the great distinction of being president of both the Royal College of Surgeons and the Royal Society, and he was appointed the first president of the General Medical Council when that august body was created in 1858.

James Syme (1799–1870), Professor of Surgery at Edinburgh, was Robert Liston's cousin and Lord Lister's father-in-law. He was a conservative surgeon who put forward the doctrine that excision of joints is usually preferable to amputation. His name is perpetuated by the term "Syme's amputation", a disarticulation of the ankle joint, in which a flap is cut from the superficial structures of the heel. It was said of him that "He never wasted a word, a drop of ink, or a drop of blood."

The leading British military surgeon of the period was George James Guthrie (1785–1856) who served in America, in the Peninsular and at Waterloo. His greatest work, his *Treatise on Gunshot Wounds* (1815), contains descriptions of war surgery which can only be compared with those of his great contemporary Baron Larrey.

Abdominal surgery had not yet come into being, but in 1837 and 1839 John Burns, surgeon to the Westminster Hospital, wrote two papers on appendicitis. He laid stress on the importance of lodgement of undigested food, fruit stones, or concretions in the caecum and appendix, and described the treatment of his day by blood-letting and the evacuation of abscesses. He stated quite definitely that acute inflammation in the right iliac region is most often caused by disease of the appendix. Dr. Thomas Addison of Guy's Hospital began about 1836 to use the term "perityphlitis" and this label became attached to a number of ill-defined abdominal conditions. Surgical treatment was still limited to the evacuation of pointing abscesses. Of special interest is a report made by Mr. Henry Hancock of Charing Cross Hospital in 1848 because it is the first record of an operation purposely designed to treat peritonitis due to inflammation of the appendix. Hancock recognized an abscess as of appendicular origin and drained it successfully, but after this more than thirty years passed before there was any further record of a similar operation.

France too had its great surgeons. Baron Larrey (1766–1842) served through all the Napoleonic wars and his fame as a military surgeon is second only to that of his great countryman Ambroise Paré. Dominique Jean Larrey was born at Baudéan near the Pyrenees. He was only thirteen when his father died, and he was educated by his uncle, who was surgeon to the General Hospital at Toulouse. After making several voyages as a ship's surgeon he went to Paris to continue his studies. In the winter of 1789 he witnessed the street fighting that ushered in the French Revolution and a large number of wounded came under his care in the Hôtel Dieu. Soon after this France was fighting for the rest of Europe and Larrey was appointed surgeon to the army of the Rhine. It was in the course of this campaign that Larrey originated first-aid to the wounded by his invention of the "flying ambulances". It was the practice at this time to station the ambulance service at the rear of the troops and to leave the wounded on the field until after the battle. Larrey went into the thick of the fight with his *ambulances volantes*, which were of two kinds: light, closed, two-wheeled vehicles for two patients, drawn by two horses for rapid transit over even ground, and heavier four-wheelers accommodating four men, drawn by four horses. The latter were for use over rough ground. The ambulances were fitted with removable litters and they carried splints, bandages, drugs and food. The flying ambulances caused a great sensation and their use soon became general in the armies of the Republic.

In 1794 Larrey first met Napoleon at Toulon and the two became fast friends. Larrey served in every one of Napoleon's campaigns in France, Germany, Spain, Italy, Egypt, Russia and Poland. He took part in no fewer than sixty battles and four hundred engagements and was thrice wounded. His life was devoted to the service of his great master and to the welfare of the wounded soldier. Under the Pyramids of Egypt and in the snows of Russia Larrey was always to the fore, a prodigy of surgical skill and an example to all in his disregard of danger and hardship. Larrey told the story of his life and campaigns in his *Mémoires de Chirurgie Militaire*, the five volumes of which contain vivid word pictures of some of the most momentous events in history. At the British attack on Alexandria, Larrey had just finished amputating the thigh of the sixty-year-old General Silly when he noticed that he was deserted by all his assistants save one and that a squadron of English cavalry was bearing down on his ambulance. He placed the general on his shoulders and ran, picking his way across a field filled with holes for the cultivation of capers, over which cavalry could not follow. Alexandria was safely reached and the general recovered.

At the Battle of Eylau which was fought in bitter cold on the surface of frozen lakes, there were 7,000 French casualties. Here Larrey displayed his remarkable powers of endurance, operating without ceasing for twenty-four hours, when the cold was so great that his assistants could not hold the instruments. He afterwards wrote: "During the whole of this action I was not conscious of the necessities of life, neither hunger, thirst, nor rest. I did not feel the cold which froze the fingers and feet of many of those around me, and my hand never lost its skill on this account." At Wagram he had a recovery rate of ninety per cent of his wounded. At the capture of Smolensk, at the beginning of the Russian campaign, he performed disarticulation of the shoulder joint on eleven men, of whom nine recovered and two died of dysentery. His speedy amputations, carried out on the field, helped to reduce sepsis. Throughout the Russian campaign he noted that the intense cold seemed to inhibit suppuration and also that it had an anaesthetic effect. Larrey's careful observations played a part in inspiring present-day work on artificial hibernation and refrigeration anaesthesia. Larrey condemned close suturing, except for facial wounds, and preferred to approximate the edges by means of adhesive plasters and bandages. In his wound treatment he excised all ragged and torn parts and removed foreign bodies and fragments of bone. He tried to minimize the amount of postoperative interference and realized the great value of immobilization.

Larrey's methods and, incidentally, the extraordinary toughness of Napoleon's troops are illustrated by the case of Colonel Lawless. This officer, the commander of the Third Foreign Regiment, had his left leg shattered by a cannon ball at the Battle of Dresden. Larrey wrote: "As I was with my light ambulance at this advanced post during the engagement, where I was in great danger, I was able to attend to him at once and amputated the leg through the tibial condyles. As the Army and the Guard were retiring on Dresden I advised this honourable patient to mount a horse again and make his way to his home in France, without stopping and without touching the dressing. I advised him simply to sponge the exterior daily and to keep the stump wrapped in a piece of cloth or sheepskin. By such measures dressings were unnecessary, especially during the season of approaching winter. My advice was followed exactly and the General [he had been promoted by this time] covered the long journey from the battlefield to his home at Tours on horseback, with his stump carried in a stirrup bandage passed over his shoulders and without having it dressed on a single occasion. On his arrival his health was generally satisfactory and on the dressing being removed the wound was healed with a linear scar." At the Battle of Borodino in 1812 Larrey either performed himself or superintended no fewer than 200 amputations in twenty-four hours. At the crossing of the Beresina in the retreat from Moscow he returned to the left bank to retrieve some surgical instruments, but was caught in the press and seemed likely to perish. He was recognized by the soldiers who picked him up and passed him over their heads to safety. Larrey continued to serve to the end. At Waterloo, after being wounded and left on the ground for dead, he was captured by the Prussians and was ordered to be shot. A Prussian Army surgeon who approached to bandage his eyes recognized Larrey, for he had attended one of his courses of lectures on surgery. The result was that Larrey was brought before von Bülow—another extraordinary trick of fate because Larrey had saved the life of von Bülow's son after the Battle of Toeplitz. The great surgeon was now treated with every consideration and was sent to Louvain, where he recovered from his wounds. After the downfall of Napoleon Larrey suffered many humiliations and was deprived of some of his offices, but the soldiers never forgot him, and the publication of his Memoirs added to his renown. He ended his days in the highest honour and repute, surviving his imperial master by twenty-one years. Napoleon, who always recognized Larrey's greatness, wrote in his will: "To the Surgeon-in-Chief of the French Army, Larrey, 100,000 francs. He is the most virtuous man I have ever known."

Guillaume Dupuytren (1777–1835), another great French surgeon, was the first to excise the lower jaw and the first to amputate the neck of the uterus for cancer. He introduced a new classification of burns, describing six degrees of severity, and devised an operation for the establishment of an artificial anus (lumbar colostomy). His name is known to every medical student by reason of his description of the peculiar deformity of the fingers known as "Dupuytren's contracture." He rose from poverty to be a Baron of the Empire and a millionaire, but his cold and overbearing manner earned for him the title of "The brigand of the Hôtel Dieu". Of his pre-eminent ability there was no question and he was universally recognized as the leading French surgeon of his day.

Some intimate glimpses of Continental surgery are given by C. B. Tilanus, a young Dutch surgeon, who kept a diary of a study tour which he made through Belgium, France and Germany in 1818–19. In Paris, Tilanus attended the clinics of Dupuytren at the Hôtel Dieu, of Alexis Boyer at the Charité, and of Baron Larrey at the Hôpital de la Garde. He reminds us of the enormous reliance that was still placed upon blood-letting at this period. Phlebotomy was resorted to in a desperate attempt to prevent the ever-present sepsis, which was regarded as being mainly caused by an impure state of the blood. The young Dutchman noted the dilemma that faced the hospital surgeon of those days: if too much blood was drawn the patient became exhausted, and if the blood-letting was stopped the inflammation increased. We are reminded too of the horrors of surgery in the pre-anaesthetic era and of the enormous mortality of operations even in the hands of such great surgeons as Dupuytren. Early in 1819 Tilanus saw Dupuytren remove a tumour from the lower jaw of a man of thirty-nine:

"One incision divides the underlip and extends to the tongue-bone; a second one, from the far side of the affected skin, joins the first incision under the chin. The flap of skin is removed, the jaw exposed and from both the sides of the gap a piece taken either by sawing until it reaches the sound bone, or broken off with bone snippers so that the distance between the two sides is now 2½ inches, and the hindmost piece now is shortened to the basis of the coronoid process. The soft portions behind the jaw are also removed where unsound, and blood-vessels tied at the same time. The operation was difficult, and took a considerable time, especially the sawing of the diseased bone, owing to inferior saws and to the absence of bone-nippers of suitable design. Lint is placed in the wound, the skin of the upper portion stitched to some extent, but the lower portion is left open for the free flow of collected saliva, pus and mucus."

And all this without any anaesthesia! On the following day the patient felt very well and had a sound sleep. There was a slight discharge tinged with blood, but no pain or swelling of any importance. Drink was given by a syringe. On the next day the patient was very weak and prostrated and he had shivering fits. He died on the thirteenth day after the operation, and, according to Tilanus, post-mortem examination did not "disclose anything of note".

An abdominal operation was an event of the greatest rarity and whenever one was to be performed it attracted a huge audience. In Boyer's clinic at the Hôpital de la Charité, Tilanus saw such an operation performed by Philibert Joseph Roux, who was Boyer's son-in-law and assistant:

"M. Roux now took the scalpel (the spectators at this time having increased to about 250 students and about 20 professional persons in the area) and having made an incision of about 3½ inches on the linea alba immediately above the pubis, soon reached the cavity of the abdomen but was not enabled until some time (perhaps about three quarters of an hour during which the patient necessarily suffered excruciating agonies) to detect, cut out and tie the diseased portion of the gut. During the whole of this difficult and appalling operation the surgeon manifested the greatest coolness and presence of mind.

"Strong ligatures armed at either end with curved needles were then passed through the thick integument in three different places along the incision. A piece of thick bougie was then placed parallel with and near to the lips of the incision on either side and the ends of the ligatures being fastened to one of them, the wound was contracted by drawing the ends attached to the other piece until the two opposing edges of the divided teguments were nearly brought together, when a pledget of lint covered with cerate was placed over the part and over that again adhesive straps and a T bandage. The patient being young and stout did not faint nor take any refreshment during the operation."

The outcome of this case is not recorded.

The real pioneer of abdominal surgery was an American surgeon, Ephraim McDowell (1771–1830), of Danville, Kentucky. Like many young American doctors of this period McDowell received part of his medical training at Edinburgh, where he took a course with John Bell. On returning to America he settled in Danville and soon acquired the reputation of being the best surgeon west of Philadelphia. Quite early in his career he became impressed with the tragic fate of women afflicted with ovarian disease. Tapping of ovarian cysts had been carried out in one or two cases, but surgery could offer no radical cure and sufferers from this condition had perforce to be left to their fate. In 1809 McDowell met with such a case of ovarian disease in his own practice and he decided to take the only course that offered any possibility of relief— indeed of life—to his patient. McDowell himself gave a vivid description of the circumstances which led him to operate:

"I was sent for in 1809 to deliver a Mrs. Crawford, near Greentown, of twins, as the two attending physicians supposed. Upon examining her vagina I soon ascertained that she was not pregnant, but had a large tumour in the abdomen which moved easily from side to side. I told the lady I could do her no good and candidly stated to her her deplorable situation; informed her that John Bell, Hunter, Hey and A. Wood, four of the first and most eminent surgeons in England and Scotland, had uniformly declared in their lectures that such was the danger of peritoneal inflammation, that opening the abdomen to extract the tumour was inevitable death. But notwithstanding this, if she thought herself prepared to die, I would take the lump from her if she would come to Danville; she came in a few days after my return home and in six days I opened her side and extracted one of the ovaria which from its diseased and enlarged state weighed upwards of twenty pounds. The intestines, as soon as the opening was made, ran out upon the table, remained out for about thirty minutes, and, being upon Christmas day, they became so cold that I thought proper to bathe them in tepid water previous to my replacing them; I then returned them, stitched up the wound, and she was perfectly well in twenty-five days."

The heroic Mrs. Crawford, who was forty-seven at the time of the operation, lived to be seventy-eight. McDowell reported this case with two others in April, 1817, following up with a report of two more cases in 1819. He performed the operation of ovariotomy thirteen times in his life and eight of his patients recovered. This master surgeon of the backwoods repeatedly performed radical operations for the cure of hernia and he carried out at least thirty-two operations for stone in the bladder without a single death. One patient upon whom he successfully operated for both stone and hernia was James K. Polk, afterwards President of the United States. McDowell was a large and vigorous man as he needed to be to stand the rigours of practice in what was then an outpost of civilization. He was also a deeply religious man and liked to operate on Sunday morning so that he could hear the prayers and hymns from the nearby church. The early years of the nineteenth century also saw the revival of blood transfusion. The hero of the revival was James Blundell (1790–1877), an obstetrician connected with Guy's and St. Thomas's Hospitals, whose professional success was such as to enable him to leave a fortune of £350,000. Blundell was stimulated to follow up the almost forgotten seventeenth-century work on transfusion by realization of his helplessness in the face of the severe and often fatal haemorrhages which sometimes ensued after childbirth. His first transfusion was, however, given to a mere man on 26 September, 1818, an historic date because this was the very first transfusion of human blood. The patient in the case was already moribund from a stomach complaint and, as no harm could be done by the experiment, Blundell decided to try out the effect of transfusion. The man received 12 to 14 ounces of blood from several donors by means of a syringe in the course of thirty to forty minutes. He temporarily improved but soon relapsed and died fifty-six hours after the transfusion. After this Blundell carried out more transfusions as occasion offered. In 1824 he recorded six attempts, nearly all of which were for excessive blood loss, but in every case transfusion had been left too late and all failed. He persevered, and in 1829 recorded in the *Lancet* a successful transfusion for post-partum haemorrhage, the patient receiving eight ounces of blood from the arm of his assistant and making a good recovery. At first Blundell used a simple form of glass syringe and cannula, sucking blood out of the donor's vein and then injecting it into the patient's vein. He then invented an instrument which he called an "Impellor" —a funnel and a pump which was fixed to the back of a chair to give it stability and also to accommodate the blood donor while blood was flowing from his arm into the funnel. He later invented a "Gravitator" for the same purpose. Blundell showed that blood was not injured by its passage through an apparatus and that the introduction of a few air bubbles into the circulation was harmless. He was not only the first to transfuse human blood into human patients, but he also established many of the fundamental points in the technique of transfusion. Following Blundell's lead one or two further blood transfusions were given in the 1820s, mostly in obstetrical cases. In one case, reported by Mr. E. Doubleday in 1825 the patient remarked after she had received six ounces of blood: "I am as strong as a bull." Nevertheless she was given a further eight ounces and with striking effect, the pulse rate falling within a short time from 140 to 104.

One or two landmarks in the subsequent history of blood transfusion may here be mentioned. Transfusion was carried out on a small scale during the American Civil War, but technical difficulties connected with premature clotting and the occurrence of accidents arising from the use of incompatible blood prevented the rapid acceptance of the process. In Germany in the 1870s an attempt was even made to revive the transfusion of lambs' blood, and when sentimental objections were raised to this method its protagonists pointed out that it was after all "only taking lamb in another form". In Britain most of the early work was carried out by obstetricians. J. H.

Aveling devised a simple apparatus for immediate transfusion. This consisted of an indiarubber tube to form a connexion between the vein of the donor and that of the recipient and a little bulb in the middle to act as an auxiliary heart. In 1872 Aveling successfully transfused a young lady of twenty-one who was dying from haemorrhage following the birth of her first baby. All other known methods of stimulation had been tried without success and the patient was sinking rapidly. She was given sixty drachms of blood from her coachman and soon recovered sufficiently to be able to remark that she was "dying". Dr. Aveling noted that "the mental improvement was not as marked and rapid as I had anticipated, but this was perhaps due to the quantity of brandy she had taken". The coachman, he was pleased to report, "was not only collected and cheerful, but able to make several useful suggestions during the process of transfusion". In spite of this and other successful cases progress was very slow. The cause of many of the untoward effects of blood transfusion were explained in 1901 when the presence of agglutinins and iso-agglutinins in the blood was demonstrated by Karl Landsteiner. In 1907 the four main blood groups were determined by Jansky of Prague. These advances were of fundamental importance and it now became possible to eliminate most of the fatalities due to incompatibility. Great progress in the application of blood transfusion was made during the First World War, one of the most important improvements being the demonstration of the anticoagulant powers of sodium citrate.

FOR FURTHER READING

Aveling, J. H. Immediate transfusion in England. *Obstet. J. Gt. Brit.*, 1873, *1*, 289.
Bailey, H. and Bishop, W. J. *Notable Names in Medicine and Surgery.* 3rd ed. 1959.
Ball, J. M. *The Sack-'em-up Men. An Account of the Rise and Fall of the Modern Resurrectionists.* 1928.
Brock, R. C. *The Life and Work of Sir Astley Cooper.* 1952.
Gordon-Taylor, Sir G. and Walls, E. W. *Sir Charles Bell, his Life and Times.* Edinburgh. 1958.
Holmes, T. *Sir Benjamin Collins Brodie.* 1898.

Jones, H. W. and Mackmull, G. The influence of James Blundell on the development of blood transfusion. *Ann. med. Hist.*, 1928, *10*, 242.

Keevil, J. J. Ralph Cuming and interscapulo-thoracic amputation in 1808. *J. Roy. Nav. med. Serv.*, 1950, *36*, 63.

Leroy-Dupré. L. A. H. *Memoir of Baron Larrey.* 1861.

Miles, A. *The Edinburgh School of Surgery before Lister.* Edinburgh. 1949.

Paterson, R. *Memorials of the Life of James Syme.* Edinburgh. 1874.

Rosen, G. An American doctor in Paris in 1828. Selections from the diary of Peter Solomon Townsend, M.D. *J. Hist. Med.*, 1951, *6*, 64.

Schachner, A. *Ephraim McDowell, "Father of Ovariotomy" and Founder of Abdominal Surgery.* Philadelphia. 1921.

Thornton, J. L. *John Abernethy, a Biography.* 1953.

Tilanus, C. B. *Surgery a Hundred Years Ago.* 1925.

Widdess, J. D. H. *A Dublin School of Medicine and Surgery.* Edinburgh. 1949.

CHAPTER NINE

The Conquest of Pain and Sepsis

IN pre-anaesthetic days operations were rushed through at lightning speed and under conditions of appalling difficulty. The most hardened surgeons had to steel themselves to perform operations which they knew would cause agony to their patients and nerve-racking distress to themselves. Even William Cheselden, who could remove a stone from the bladder in under a minute, said that he had bought his reputation dearly, "for no one ever endured more anxiety and sickness before an operation". Sir Astley Cooper confessed that "he felt too much before he began ever to make a perfect operator".

As we have seen, the use of soporific potions goes back to remote antiquity and there are many references in early medical writings to pain-killing drugs given by mouth or by inhalation from a saturated sponge. Doubts have been expressed about the efficacy of many of these preparations and we have no real evidence as to the extent to which they were actually used. That they were used occasionally would seem to be highly probable, because, apart from the statements of medical writers, there are a number of references to the use of soporifics in general literature. One of the most interesting of these occurs in Boccaccio's *Decameron*, which was written in the middle of the fourteenth century:

> "It happened that there came to the attention of the physician a patient with a gangrenous leg, and when the master had made an examination he told the relatives that unless a decayed bone in the leg were removed either the entire leg would have to be amputated or the patient die; moreover, if the bone were removed, the patient might recover, but he refused to undertake the case except as if the man were already dead. To this the relatives agreed and surrendered the patient to him.
>
> "The doctor was of opinion that without an opiate the

man could not endure the pain and would not permit the operation, and since the affair was set for the evening, he distilled that morning a type of water after his own composition which had the faculty of bringing to the person who drank it sleep for as long a time as was deemed necessary to complete the operation."

The almost complete absence of any mention of pain-relieving drugs in medical literature of the post-medieval period is not easy to explain. It is, however, probable that the action of the crude concoctions used in early times was very uncertain, and that drugged sleep often ended in death. The active ingredients of the many herbs used in medicine had not of course been isolated and it would have been very difficult to regulate dosages. The case is somewhat similar to that of blood transfusion, with which there was also a very long gap between the first trials and the successful application of the method in practice.

One method of producing analgesia that seems to have been used intermittently from quite early times was compression. Writing in 1564 about the various uses of the tourniquet Ambroise Paré states that "it much dulls the sense of the part by stupefying it". In 1784 James Carrick Moore, a young London surgeon, published a pamphlet on *A Method of Preventing or Diminishing Pain in several Operations of Surgery*. His idea was to blunt the sensibility of nerves by compressing them with a screw tourniquet of his own design. Moore refers to the use of anodynes, the most powerful of which was opium; but he says that the largest dose he ventured to give had little or no effect in lessening the sufferings of the patient during operation. He communicated his views to John Hunter, and that great surgeon, ever ready to encourage young men with ideas, used Moore's "Compressor" when operating on one of his patients in St. George's Hospital. The case was one of amputation below the knee, and the patient said afterwards that although his sufferings were greatly diminished the tying of a small bleeding vessel gave him great pain. It was apparently decided that the result did not warrant any further trial of Moore's apparatus and no more was heard of it.

The next step in the search for a satisfactory method of inducing surgical anaesthesia is connected with the earliest scientific work on hypnotism. The pioneers of hypnotism were in turn inspired by the pseudo-science of mesmerism or animal magnetism which had been exploited by Franz Anton Mesmer (1734–1815). Mesmer was generally derided as a quack, but he had studied medicine and was in fact one of the earliest exponents of psychotherapy. His ideas were taken up by two British investigators, who laid the foundations of modern hypnotism. James Braid, a Scottish surgeon who had settled in Manchester, became interested in the subject of animal magnetism about 1841. He proved that the mesmeric influence is entirely subjective or personal and that no fluid or electricity passes from the operator to the patient. In 1843 he published a book on the subject entitled *Neurypnology or the Rationale of Nervous Sleep*. Contemporaneously with Braid, Dr. John Elliotson, of University College Hospital, began to study the applications of hypnotism and in 1843 he published a pamphlet describing *Numerous Cases of Surgical Operations without Pain in the Mesmeric State*. The views of both Braid and Elliotson met with violent opposition from two sides: they were denounced by their medical colleagues as charlatans and were bitterly opposed by the professional mesmerists who wished to exploit the method as something supernatural. Elliotson was forced to resign his post of professor of medicine in the University of London. Two years after this James Esdaile, a Scottish surgeon in the service of the East India Company, read Elliotson's pamphlet, and, although he had never seen anyone mesmerized, decided to use the method for the purpose of preventing pain during a surgical operation. On 4 April, 1845, Esdaile had to carry out two extremely painful operations upon a middle-aged Hindu convict. When the pain was most severe and only one operation had been completed he tried to soothe the patient by the "mesmeric passes". He persevered in his attempt and after some time induced a condition of deep sleep in which his patient was quite indifferent to pinpricks and other painful stimuli. A week later Esdaile mesmerized the same patient before the second operation and when the Hindu awoke thirteen hours later he was quite unaware that anything had been done to him. An account of this experiment was given by Esdaile in a medical journal but his colleagues regarded him as an easily duped enthusiast. Esdaile continued to mesmerize his patients and within a year he had successfully performed 100 operations under its influence. His results were reported to the Government and a committee was appointed by the deputy-governor of Bengal to investigate the subject. The committee drew up a very favourable report and recommended that every help should be given to the enterprising surgeon. A small hospital in Calcutta was placed at Esdaile's disposal and he eventually had a record of 261 painless operations with a mortality of 5.5 per cent. All this work was fully described in his book, *Mesmerism in India*, published in 1846. In 1851 Esdaile returned to his native Scotland and there he died in 1859 at the age of fifty. He tried some hypnotic experiments in Scotland but found that his hard-headed countrymen were far less impressionable than Hindus and that it was very often difficult to place them in a deep hypnotic trance.

The further development of anaesthesia by means of hypnotism was inhibited by two factors. In the first place, not all patients were equally susceptible and induction of an hypnotic trance sufficiently deep to guarantee insensibility to pain took a very long time. Secondly, the work of Elliotson, Braid and Esdaile coincided in time with that of the early pioneers of ether anaesthesia. Two entirely different methods of preventing pain during surgical operations were developing at the same time.

The story of inhalation anaesthesia begins in 1799 when Sir Humphry Davy recorded the effects produced by the inhalation of nitrous oxide. He himself breathed various concentrations of the pure gas and noted that a headache and the pain associated with the cutting of a wisdom tooth were relieved. In 1800 he suggested that the gas might "probably be used with advantage in surgical operations in which no great effusion of blood takes place". Sir Humphrey was not a medical man and his hint was not followed up at that time. Demonstrations of the effects of nitrous oxide were frequently given, bladders filled with "laughing gas" being passed round at lectures.

The inhalation of nitrous oxide even became a popular party game. A little book of 1839 contains a description of the "irresistibly ridiculous" sight of a large room filled with persons each of whom was sucking from a bladder. As the gas began to take effect "some jumped over the tables and chairs; some were bent on making speeches; some were very much inclined to fight; and one young gentleman persisted in attempting to kiss the ladies". At about the same time "ether frolics" became equally popular.

The first attempt to eliminate the pain of a surgical operation by the inhalation of a gas was made by a young surgeon named Henry Hill Hickman. In 1823 Hickman attempted to bring about a state of "suspended animation" in animals by means of carbon dioxide. In 1824 he published a plea for the use of "suspended animation" in surgical operations and gave details of his experiments. It seems that he never tried his method on a human subject and his work had no influence on susbsequent developments. Hickman's death in 1830, at the early age of thirty and before he could follow up his novel ideas, was a tragedy.

The early history of the introduction of anaesthesia has been the subject of much controversy, but the principal facts are now well established. In January 1842 William E. Clarke, a young physician of Rochester, U.S.A., who had acquired some knowledge of ether by attendance at "ether frolics", administered ether on a towel to a Miss Hobbie who then had one of her teeth extracted painlessly. So far as is known this was the first use of ether for a dental or surgical operation, but Clarke does not seem to have realized the importance of his discovery and he made no attempt to follow it up.

On 30 March, 1842, Dr. Crawford W. Long of Danielsville, Georgia, who had also witnessed some ether frolics, successfully removed a small tumour from the neck of a patient under the influence of ether. During the next few years Long gave ether in other cases and claims have been made for him as the discoverer of anaesthesia. Statues have been erected in his honour and he is also commemorated on a United States postage stamp. It was not until 1849, however, that Long published anything about his use of ether and long before that time surgical anaesthesia had been publicly demonstrated and had spread to all parts of the world.

The next contestant for the title of the "discoverer" of anaesthesia was Horace Wells, a dentist of Hartford, Connecticut, who, on 10 December, 1844, attended a public demonstration of the effects of nitrous oxide. On the following day he decided to try the effect of nitrous oxide for tooth extraction and had one of his own teeth pulled out by a colleague. Wells exclaimed after this: "I didn't feel it so much as the prick of a pin." After giving nitrous oxide in several further cases, Wells went to Boston, where he was asked to give a demonstration in the Harvard medical school. The demonstration was duly given in January 1845, but unfortunately the boy whose tooth was being extracted groaned during the operation, although he later stated that he had felt no pain. The critical audience laughed and from Wells's point of view the demonstration was a dismal failure. Wells returned to Hartford and continued to use nitrous oxide, but one of his cases ended fatally and this caused him to withdraw from practice. He eventually took his own life. In the meantime William Thomas Green Morton, another dentist, who had been a pupil of Wells and had witnessed the unsuccessful demonstration in January 1845, was experimenting with various substances. On 30 September, 1836, Morton made use of sulphuric ether, the anaesthetic properties of which had been pointed out to him by Dr. Charles T. Jackson, a well-known chemist, for the extraction of a deeply-rooted tooth. Morton then visited Dr. John Collins Warren, one of the surgeons of the Massachusetts General, and asked permission to give ether in a surgical case. Permission was given and on 16 October, 1846, Morton administered the new anaesthetic while Dr. Warren removed a tumour from the neck of a young man named Gilbert Abbott. The demonstration was completely successful, and as the patient came back to consciousness Warren turned to the excited audience of students and exclaimed, "Gentlemen, this is no humbug." On the following day Morton again gave sulphuric ether and Dr. Hayward removed a large fatty tumour of the shoulder. In his next case Morton was unable to anaesthetize the patient, but on November 7 he had another spectacular success with an operation for the amputation of a leg. On 18 November, 1846, the great discovery was announced to the world in a paper by Dr. Henry J. Bigelow, published in the *Boston Medical and Surgical Journal*. Morton probably has the best claim to be regarded as the discoverer of surgical anaesthesia, but his conduct subsequent to the Boston demonstrations was in marked contrast to that of the eminent surgeons who had given him his opportunity. He tried to patent his discovery and spent the rest of his life trying to establish his claims.

News of the successful operations performed at Boston spread with remarkable rapidity. On 28 November, 1846, Professor Jacob Bigelow (father of Henry J. Bigelow) wrote a letter to his friend, Dr. Francis Boott, of Gower Street, London, telling him about Morton's achievements. Dr. Boott communicated the news to his friend James Robinson, a dentist, who on December 19 successfully carried out a dental extraction while Boott administered ether. Meanwhile Boott had also written to Robert Liston, the celebrated surgeon, of University College Hospital, and on December 21, Liston carried out the first major operation under anaesthesia in Europe—an amputation of the thigh. Everything went well and at the conclusion of the operation Liston is supposed to have remarked, "Gentlemen, this Yankee dodge beats mesmerism hollow."

By February 1847 the *Lancet* and other medical journals were reporting anaesthetic operations from all parts of Great Britain and ether had already been used in most European countries. Within four months news of the Boston operations had reached the Cape of Good Hope direct from America and on 16 June, 1847, a leg was painlessly amputated by Dr. W. G. Atherstone of Grahamstown. No details of Morton's method of administering ether had been received and Dr. Atherstone appears to have been unaware of the London operations. He was forced to improvise his own anaesthetic apparatus from a large bottle with a cork that had two holes in it for the passage of tubes—the whole thing somewhat resembling a Turkish hubble-bubble. With this crude apparatus the patient was rendered insensible and his leg was removed without his being conscious of anything. When he came round he did not know what had happened and could not believe that his leg had really been removed. "What? My leg off? Impossible—I can't believe it—let me see for myself. (And on seeing the stump he burst out:) God be praised! It's the greatest discovery ever made!"

In January 1847 James Young Simpson of Edinburgh was the first to use ether as an anaesthetic in midwifery practice; but as this drug had several drawbacks, not least of which was its smell, he carried out a number of experiments upon himself and his friends with a view to discovering a better general anaesthetic. One evening Simpson and his friends tried the effect of inhaling chloroform (which had been discovered in 1831-2) and they all became unconscious. When Simpson recovered consciousness his colleagues were still lying helpless under the table and he realized that he had hit upon an anaesthetic that was far stronger than ether. On 10 November, 1847, Simpson read his "Account of a new anaesthetic agent" to the Edinburgh Medico-Chirurgical Society, and five days later he administered chloroform while Professor James Miller operated on a boy suffering from osteomyelitis of the radius. As is well known, there was at first intense opposition to the use of chloroform in midwifery on theological grounds, but Simpson reminded his opponents that the Lord caused a deep sleep to fall on Adam before the birth of Eve and opposition virtually ceased when Queen Victoria consented to the use of chloroform in her own case in 1853.

By the middle of the nineteenth century pain had been banished from surgical operations, but one grave danger still faced every patient submitting himself to the surgeon's knife. This was the ever-present risk of sepsis. Hospital diseases—erysipelas, pyaemia, septicaemia and gangrene—were rife. That all these diseases were due to some form of "contagion" had long been suspected, but the general view was that whatever was responsible for the contagion or infection was generated spontaneously in wounds. Alternatively it was thought that air itself was the agent responsible for suppuration and many attempts were made to exclude the air from wounds by means of elaborate dressings.

Some medical men had postulated the existence of minute particles in the air which carried "contagion". The Italian Girolamo Fracastoro had in 1546 even referred to "seminaria, the seeds of disease which multiply rapidly and propagate their life". In his treatise *De Contagione* he described three modes of infection—by contact, by clothing, utensils, etc., and infection at a distance by the air. One of the difficulties that made the doctrine of contagion difficult of acceptance was that no one could see the supposed particles or agents. Magnifying lenses were used in ancient times, and by the beginning of the seventeenth century they had been combined in a tube to form the compound microscope. The first man to employ the microscope in investigating the causes of diseases was probably Athanasius Kircher, a learned Jesuit priest. In 1658 Kircher described experiments upon the nature of putrefaction, showing how maggots and other living creatures developed in decaying matter. He also claimed to have found in the blood of plague-stricken patients "countless masses of small worms, invisible to the naked eye". It is impossible that he could have seen the plague bacillus with the very low-power microscopes at his disposal, and it is generally believed that his "worms" were pus cells or blood corpuscles. Nevertheless, he may have seen some of the larger micro-organisms and his statements about the doctrine of contagion are even more explicit than those of Fracastoro. The great pioneer of modern microscopy was Anthony van Leeuwenhoek, a Dutch linen draper, who ground his own lenses and made hundreds of microscopes. Leeuwenhoek devoted his leisure to microscopical studies, the results of which he communicated to the Royal Society in London. Few of his instruments provided a magnification of more than 160 but they enabled him to make many discoveries of the greatest importance. Leeuwenhoek was the first to describe spermatozoa and he gave the first complete account of the red blood corpuscles. He found that the film from his own teeth contained "little animals, more numerous than all the people in the Netherlands".

In spite of the prophetic utterings of Fracastoro and Kircher and of the observations of Leeuwenhoek and other early microscopists, medical men were very slow to accept the theory of infection by micro-organisms. Even those who were disposed to believe in the existence of disease-causing organisms were misled by the theory of "spontaneous generation". According to this theory the small forms of life that appeared in decaying matter could arise by themselves—that is to say they had no living parents. This doctrine was combated even in the seventeenth century but it was not finally disposed of until the time of Pasteur and Lister. From the medical point of view the important fact about the doctrine of spontaneous generation was that those who believed in it could not see the necessity for the strict exclusion of contagion from without. Brief reference must be made to one or two investigators who came very near to the discovery of the antiseptic principle.

As early as 1795 Dr. Alexander Gordon of Aberdeen had advised that "nurses and physicians attending patients affected with puerperal fever ought to wash themselves and get their apparel properly fumigated". In 1843 Dr. Oliver Wendell Holmes, Professor of Anatomy at Harvard—but better known for his delightful "Breakfast Table" essays—read a paper "On the Contagiousness of Puerperal Fever". He affirmed the contagious nature of the disease and laid down rigorous rules for its prevention by washing of hands and changing of clothing.

Further proof of the contagious nature of puerperal fever was provided by Ignaz Philipp Semmelweis, an assistant in the maternity hospital at Vienna. At this hospital the mortality rate among women after childbirth reached the appalling figure of ten per cent. In investigating these deaths from puerperal fever Semmelweis noticed that the appearances after death were the same as those observed in the body of one of his colleagues who had died of a dissection wound. Semmelweis came to the correct conclusion that all the deaths were caused by infection from "putrid material", carried on the hands of students who often went direct from the dissecting room to the labour wards. Semmelweis instituted a routine of hand-washing with chloride of lime and by this simple measure the mortality was reduced to 1.27 per cent. The ideas of Semmelweis met with fierce opposition and he left Vienna in disgust. His fate was tragic: the neglect of his work so preyed on his sensitive mind that he became insane and he died in 1865 at the age of forty-seven.

The work of these pioneers in the field of obstetrics had no immediate repercussions in surgical practice. Simple methods of disinfection were sometimes effective, but the problem was still obscure and the antiseptic system still lacked a proper scientific basis.

The man who elucidated the true nature of infection, founded the science of bacteriology, and paved the way for Lister and the antiseptic system in surgery was Louis Pasteur (1822–95).

Pasteur was led to his great discoveries regarding bacteria and other micro-organisms by his investigations into the process of fermentation. Up to the time of Pasteur the fermentation of wine had been regarded as being caused by the spontaneous generation of some noxious agents or by purely chemical means. Pasteur showed conclusively that fermentation was brought about by some agent which entered the wine from without. He proved by painstaking experiments under rigorously controlled conditions that meat and fluids like blood did not putrefy if they were kept in such a way that all air was excluded from them. By taking samples of air at different levels Pasteur showed that contamination became less with increasing altitude. Then he proved that the contaminating agents were living organisms (bacteria) which were everywhere—in every room, in the air, on every article of clothing, on furniture, on the ground, and on the skin. He showed that putrefaction was caused by the presence of bacteria and that this applied to putrefaction in foods and in wounds. Pasteur next showed that certain diseases were caused by micro-organisms and he devised means of preventing these diseases by the use of vaccines, prepared from attenuated or weakened cultures of the organisms in question. Pasteur's greatest triumphs were in regard to the causation and prevention of anthrax and rabies but the principles of his revolutionary discoveries were soon extended to many other diseases, for example, diphtheria, typhoid fever, cholera and plague.

The application of Pasteur's discoveries to surgical practice was the work of Joseph Lister, a young English surgeon whose character and achievements give him a place among the very greatest names in medicine. As a young medical student Lister had been present at the first operation under ether anaesthesia by Robert Liston at University College Hospital in December 1846. In 1860 he was appointed professor of surgery at Glasgow at a critical period in the history of medicine. The introduction of anaesthesia had made more operations possible—surgeons were beginning to open the abdomen— but the mortality of operations performed in hospitals became greater than ever before. Sir James Young Simpson, the celebrated obstetrician who introduced chloroform, said that "A man laid on an operating table in one of our surgical hospitals is exposed to more chances of death than was the English soldier on the field of Waterloo". This was in fact an understatement. In the 1850s the death rate after amputations varied from 25 to 60 per cent in different countries and in military practice it reached the appalling figure of 75 to 90 per cent. The earliest ovariotomies, which were the first abdominal operations performed on a fairly large scale, had a mortality rate of more than 30 per cent even in the most expert hands.

Some attempt at cleanliness was made by the early nineteenth-century surgeons—for example, a surgeon usually kept a special coat for operating or he even wore an apron, but these garments were often stiff with congealed blood and matter. Surgeons sometimes washed their hands and cleaned their instruments—but often *after* rather than before operating.

As a young hospital surgeon Lister was appalled by the frightful results of even the most simple of operations and he devoted much time to the study of inflammation and suppuration. While he was working on the problem his colleague, Thomas Anderson, the Professor of Chemistry, drew his attention to the work of Louis Pasteur who had, as we have already seen, shown that putrefaction was a fermentation caused by microscopic organisms carried in the air and on dust. Lister applied Pasteur's principles to the prevention of suppuration. He determined to prevent the access of organisms by killing them in or on the surface of the wound. After trying various chemical agents he finally selected carbolic acid and he insisted that everything which touched the wound, the dressings, the instruments and the fingers, should be treated with this antiseptic. He even produced an antiseptic atmosphere by means of a carbolic spray.

The antiseptic system was first used by Lister in 1865 in a case of compound fracture of the leg. In 1867 he published his first results: eleven cases, nine recoveries of life and limb, one amputation, and one death. These results were maintained and Lister published detailed descriptions of his methods. He applied the antiseptic principle to such conditions as abscesses in the spine and the joints, and operations on the breast. In 1869 Lister succeeded his father-in-law, James Syme, in the chair of surgery at Edinburgh and in 1877 he accepted the post of Professor of Surgery at King's College, London. Long before his retirement from practice in 1896 his fame was world-wide. In 1897 he became the first medical man to be raised to the peerage. The character of Lister matched his powers as an original investigator and as a practical surgeon. He never lost an opportunity of acknowledging his indebtedness to Pasteur. In his first letter to the great French savant written in 1874 he wrote: "Allow me to take this opportunity to tender you my most cordial thanks for having, by your brilliant researches, demonstrated to me the truth of the germ theory of putrefaction, and thus furnished me with the principle upon which alone the antiseptic system can be carried out." And in 1902, almost at the end of his long life, he wrote: "All efforts to combat decomposition of the blood in open wounds were in vain until Pasteur's researches opened a new way, by combating the microbes."

As so frequently happens, Lister's views were accepted and their value was recognized abroad sooner than at home. One of his earliest supporters was Professor Saxtorph, of Copenhagen, who as early as 1870 wrote to tell Lister that he had banished sepsis from his wards by antiseptic methods. German surgeons played a very important part in the adoption of the antiseptic system. They, like their colleagues in all countries, had been appalled at the prevalence of sepsis in their wards. Hospital gangrene was so rife in Halle that it was said that no one dared to touch a knife in the surgical clinic. This frightful state of affairs was altered by Richard von Volkmann, who was appointed Professor of Surgery at Halle in 1867, the year in which Lister published his first paper on the antiseptic system. Volkmann studied all Lister's writings and he became his most powerful advocate in Germany. The antiseptic ritual was carried out in every detail, as appears from a vivid description of Volkmann's clinic left by a British surgeon who visited it in 1879. All wounds were irrigated freely with 1-in-20 carbolic lotion, while the "donkey engine" or spray filled the air with antiseptic vapour. The surgeon and his assistants wore long rubber boots and as soon as Volkmann called "watering can", carbolic lotion was poured out from gardeners' watering cans with long spouts. The slogan of the clinic was: "If dirt be unavoidable, it must be antiseptic dirt".

The Franco-Prussian war provided a wonderful opportunity for the trial of Lister's methods. In 1872 the German hospitals were crowded with soldiers suffering from severely infected wounds. At Leipzig and at Halle the results of Listerism were almost magical: pyaemia was banished and there was a dramatic fall in the death rate. Very striking was the experience of Professor von Nussbaum of Munich. At his hospital in 1872 eighty per cent of all wounds were affected by pyaemia and gangrene and the death rate was terrifying. The antiseptic method was introduced and within a week von Nussbaum was able to report: "Not another case of hospital gangrene appeared. . . . Our results become better and better, the time of healing shorter, and pyaemia and erysipelas completely disappear." Anxious to spread the gospel of Listerism, Nussbaum wrote in 1875 a little book on the antiseptic treatment of wounds which passed through many editions in various languages.

In 1876 Lucas Championnière of Paris, who had visited Lister in Glasgow in order to study his methods, also published a book on antiseptic surgery. Professor Ernst von Bergmann of Berlin was mainly responsible for the introduction of the "aseptic method", which was simply another means of applying the principles so clearly stated by Lister. Antisepsis and asepsis are simply different aspects of the same thing. The results were equally good if all micro-organisms were killed

or if they were entirely excluded from the scene of the operation. Von Bergmann tried to make his operating theatre
germ-free. In 1886 he introduced steam sterilization of towels,
gowns and dressings. Gustav Neuber of Kiel built a private
hospital which was planned for the express purpose of carrying
out the aseptic technique. "Dirty" cases were completely
separated from "clean" cases by the use of five operating
theatres. The air of the theatres was sterilized by heat and by
passing it through a cotton filter. In his book on aseptic wound
treatment published in 1886 Neuber stressed many other
points. These included disinfection of the skin of the patient;
the surgeon and his assistants to go through a ritual washing
and to wear sterilized caps, aprons and rubber boots; the instruments and accessories to be sterilized by boiling and then placed
in carbolic acid solution; wounds to be irrigated with a weak
solution of mercuric chloride and a sterile dressing applied;
the number of spectators was limited and they were all forced
to undergo the same preparation as the operating team.

Some British surgeons who were contemporary with Lister
achieved remarkable results, although the antiseptic system
came too late to have much effect upon their techniques. The
greatest operator at the middle of the century was Sir William
Fergusson, Professor of Surgery at King's College, London.
Fergusson was a pupil of Dr. Robert Knox of Edinburgh and
under the tuition of that great anatomist he became a first-
class dissector. All contemporary accounts agree as to his
superlative skill as an operator. He had large and powerful
hands and when the nature of the operation called for speed
he was extraordinarily quick. It was said that if you blinked
when he was cutting for stone in the bladder or amputating
a leg you might see no operation at all. His assistants were
expected to remain absolutely silent while he was operating
and he himself never spoke until the patient was off the
table. Some of his greatest successes were in the surgical
correction of harelip and cleft palate. Out of 134 cases of
cleft palate upon which he operated between 1828 and 1864
he was able to claim 129 successes, and among 400 cases of
harelip operated upon by him during the same period there
were only three failures. Fergusson invented many instruments,

the best known of which are his lion forceps, speculum, and mouth gag. With all his confidence and skill he never operated unless operation was imperatively demanded and he never did more than was absolutely necessary. It was he, in fact, who coined the term "conservative surgery".

Another great conservative surgeon, Sir James Paget, of St. Bartholomew's Hospital, is remembered for his original descriptions of Paget's disease of bone and Paget's disease of the breast. He was a sound but not a brilliant operator, his forte being diagnosis. Sir James Paget became President of the Royal College of Surgeons and Serjeant-Surgeon to the Queen. He was an admirable teacher and writer and was regarded as one of the most eloquent speakers of his day. So great a judge as Mr. Gladstone said that he divided people into two classes—those who had, and those who had not, heard James Paget.

Sir Jonathan Hutchinson, a Quaker like Lister, was another noted President of the Royal College of Surgeons. He was surgeon to the London Hospital and of Moorefields Eye Hospital. His name is commemorated in the terms "Hutchinson's teeth" and "Hutchinson's pupils"—the first being one of the signs of congenital syphilis and the second being associated with traumatic haemorrhage within the skull. Hutchinson wrote voluminously on every aspect of surgery and was indeed described as a "universal specialist". He was a life-long collector and after his retirement to Haslemere in Surrey he founded the Haslemere Educational Museum which is still open to the public.

James Marion Sims was a brilliant American surgeon whose career began in the days before anaesthesia and antisepsis. As early as 1835 he operated successfully for abscess of the liver and in 1837 removed both the upper and lower jaw of a patient. In 1878 he performed the operation of cholecystostomy for drainage of the gall bladder. Sims is, however, best known for his achievements as a gynaecological surgeon. In 1852 he devised an operation which revolutionized the treatment of vesico-vaginal fistula, a very troublesome condition which had hitherto resisted all attempts at operative treatment. Henry Jacob Bigelow of Boston was the first American to excise the hip joint (1852) and he devised an ingenious method of crushing and removing stones of the bladder (1878).

FOR FURTHER READING

Burrows, E. H. The first anaesthetic in South Africa. *Med. Hist.*, 1958, *2*, 47.

Duncum, B. *The Development of Inhalation Anaesthesia.* 1947.

Godlee, Sir R. *Lord Lister.* 3rd ed. Oxford. 1924.

Guthrie, D. *Lord Lister, his Life and Doctrine.* Edinburgh. 1949.

Hutchinson, H. *Jonathan Hutchinson: Life and Letters.* 1946.

Keys, T. E. *The History of Surgical Anaesthesia.* New York. 1945.

Paget, Sir J. *Memoirs and Letters of Sir James Paget.* 1901.

Plarr, V. G. *Lives of the Fellows of the Royal College of Surgeons of England.* 2 vols. 1930.

Porter, I. A. *Alexander Gordon, M.D., of Aberdeen, 1752–1799.* Edinburgh. 1958.

Sims, J. M. *The Story of My Life.* New York. 1884.

Sinclair, Sir W. J. *Semmelweis, his Life and Doctrine.* Manchester. 1909.

Thomas, K. B. John Hunter and an amputation under analgesia in 1784. *Med. Hist.*, 1958, *2*, 53.

Underwood, E. A. Before and after Morton. A historical survey of anaesthesia. *Brit. Med. J.*, 1946, *ii*, 525.

Vallery-Radot, P. *The Life of Louis Pasteur.* 2 vols. 1902.

CHAPTER TEN

Surgery after Lister

THE introduction of anaesthesia and antisepsis enabled surgeons to carry out procedures that had formerly been quite beyond them, including long operations within the head, the abdomen and the pelvis. First among the founders of modern abdominal surgery stands Theodor Billroth of Vienna. In 1872 this great surgeon resected the oesophagus, in 1878 parts of the intestines, and in 1881 the pyloric end of the stomach. He also made the first complete excision of the larynx. His pupil, Anton Woelfler, introduced the operation of gastro-enterostomy— the creation of an artificial passage between the stomach and the intestines.

Richard von Volkmann of Halle was in 1878 the first to excise the rectum for cancer. He was a bold and elegant operator and surgeons flocked to his clinic from all parts of Europe. Volkmann was one of the first to draw attention to the fact that cancer of the skin can arise from constant exposure to irritating substances, such as certain oils. Friedrich von Esmarch, professor of surgery at Kiel, greatly advanced military surgery. He was the inventor of Esmarch's rubber bandage which, when properly applied, allows operations to be carried out on the lower limbs through a bloodless field. His extensive war service had convinced him of the necessity of first-aid on the battlefield and he advised that every soldier should carry a first-aid outfit and should be instructed in its use. His book, *First Aid to the Injured*, published in 1875, became the best-known work on the subject. Esmarch was an uncle by marriage of the Emperor William II and he enjoyed the title of Excellency.

Karl Thiersch, Professor of Surgery at Erlangen and Leipzig, was one of the German pioneers of Listerism. He revolutionized the practice of modern plastic surgery by his invention of the Thiersch skin graft, which he described at a meeting of the

German Surgical Society in 1874. Gustav Simon, of Rostock and Heidelberg, was a pioneer in the surgery of the kidney and was in 1869 the first to excise that organ. He also wrote on excision of the spleen and on plastic surgery.

Johann von Mikulicz-Radecki, a Pole by birth, became Professor of Surgery at Königsberg and Breslau. He greatly extended the operative surgery of the stomach and the joints, and was one of the first surgeons to wear cotton gloves when operating. It seems that the gloves were worn in order to secure a firmer grip on the instruments rather than with the idea of preventing infection. However that may be, they were soon superseded by rubber gloves, which were introduced by William Stewart Halsted, surgeon to the Johns Hopkins Hospital at Baltimore, in 1889-90. Curiously enough the use of rubber gloves had been suggested by Sir Thomas Watson, a physician, in 1843—long before the days of antisepsis—but the idea was not followed up. According to Halsted's own account he was led to experiment with rubber gloves after the nurse in charge of his operating room had complained that the mercuric chloride used as a disinfectant produced a dermatitis of her hands and arms. "As she was an unusually efficient woman," said Halsted, "I gave the matter my consideration and one day in New York requested the Goodyear Rubber Company to make as an experiment two pairs of thin rubber gloves with gauntlets. On trial they proved so satisfactory that additional gloves were ordered." By 1896 the wearing of gloves by all concerned in the operation had become a regular part of the Johns Hopkins technique. As a postscript to this story, it may be added that the nurse in the case became Mrs. Halsted.

Halsted also introduced gutta-percha tissue for drainage purposes and silver foil dressings. He was a wonderfully successful operator and he advanced almost every department of surgery. Among his most important achievements was the introduction of the modern operation for the radical cure of hernia and his method of radical mastectomy—one of the greatest contributions ever made to the treatment of cancer of the breast. Halsted also carried out the first experiments on local infiltration anaesthesia with cocaine.

The control of haemorrhage still posed problems for the surgeon, especially during the performance of the long abdominal operations that were now possible. The modern artery clamp was introduced by Eugène Koeberle of Alsace and Jules Péan of Paris in 1862. These two surgeons were, incidentally, among the first on the Continent to perform ovariotomy, and Péan in 1879 was the first to remove the stomach for cancer. A further great improvement in the control of haemorrhage was made by Sir Thomas Spencer Wells of London. Wells was originally a naval surgeon, but he decided to specialize in gynaecological surgery and in 1854 was elected surgeon to the Samaritan Hospital for Women in London. He interrupted his career to serve during the Crimean War and gained considerable experience of gunshot wounds. On his return to London Wells became greatly interested in the operation of ovariotomy, which was then being performed by a few bold surgeons in the face of the bitterest opposition from the majority of their colleagues. Initially, the results of the operation were appalling and those who continued to attempt it were denounced as murderers. Wells was determined to change this and he persisted on the course which he had mapped out. In 1858 he performed his first successful ovariotomy. By his superb skill and by meticulous attention to detail he turned the operation into one of comparative safety, and in 1880 he was able to publish an account of his first 1,000 cases. The original Spencer Wells forceps were introduced in January 1874. They were based upon the old artery forceps of Robert Liston and the crude "bulldog" forceps of the famous German surgeon, J. F. Dieffenbach. Spencer Wells forceps—slightly modified from their original form—are now used in every hospital and clinic in the world.

Robert Lawson Tait enjoyed even greater success as an abdominal surgeon than Spencer Wells. He numbered his successful cases by the thousand and was a pioneer in almost every phase of gynaecological surgery. Strangely enough Spencer Wells did not adopt the antiseptic method until late in his career, and Lawson Tait always remained a violent opponent of Listerism. The secret of their success, apart from their extraordinary skill, was their attention to cleanliness.

Wells made liberal use of soap and water and Lawson Tait boiled his instruments and his ligatures although he scorned the use of antiseptics. The success achieved by the ovariotomists led to a great extension of abdominal surgery.

Curiously enough, removal of the appendix, now the commonest of all abdominal operations, did not become common until the very end of the century. An important landmark was the paper of the American Willard Parker who, in 1867, recognized three important stages of acute appendicitis—gangrene, perforating ulcer, and abscess. He described four successful operations for the drainage of abscesses and defined a period between the fifth and the twelfth day of the disease as the optimal time for incision. Willard Parker's paper did much to encourage operation for perityphlitic abscesses, for in the next fifteen years some 80 cases of operation were recorded. During this time the clinical history of the condition was being studied and careful post-mortem examinations were indicating the true origin of perityphlitic abscesses.

In 1884 Samuel Fenwick, physician to the London Hospital, advised early operation for appendicitis, writing as follows: "A disease of rare occurrence, which has only of late years attracted the attention of practitioners, and which often presents considerable difficulty in diagnosis, viz., perforation of the vermiform appendix. Five cases of this kind have been admitted into the hospital during the last twelve months . . . theoretically it would seem to be much better if we could cut down upon the appendix as soon as the diagnosis was tolerably certain, and remove from its neighbourhood any concretion or decomposing material that might be the cause of the irritation."

Dr. Fenwick's excellent advice met with little response in Great Britain although Sir Charters Symonds operated at Guy's Hospital about this time upon a twenty-three-year-old man suffering from "recurrent typhlitis", removing a calculus from a much twisted appendix.

One of the most famous of the brilliant band of surgeons who laid the foundations of the modern knowledge of appendicitis was Reginald Heber Fitz of Boston. Fitz laid down rules for treatment which had an enormous influence in the development of the surgical attack on the condition. His epoch-making paper on "Perforating inflammation of the vermiform appendix, with special reference to its early diagnosis and treatment" was read at the first meeting of the Association of American Physicians in 1886. Fitz clearly outlined the main symptoms of the disease and coined the name by which it has always been known since 1886—"As a circumscribed peritonitis is simply one event, although usually the most important, in the history of inflammation of the appendix, it seems preferable to use the term *appendicitis* to express the primary condition." Fitz emphasized that the chief danger was perforation. "In the light of our present knowledge," he wrote, "the surgical treatment of this lesion offers the best chances for the life and future of the patient, and the progress of the disease needs to be watched with knife in hand."

In 1884 the great German surgeon Johann von Mikulicz advocated the treatment of all types of perforation of the gastro-intestinal tract by urgent laparotomy. About this time he dealt with a case of general peritonitis due to a perforated appendix. In this case Mikulicz failed to locate the appendix but he realized that he might have saved the patient's life had he been able to find and remove the gangrenous organ. He therefore recommended that the acutely inflamed appendix should be removed. The first recorded attempt to carry out Mikulicz's suggestion was apparently made by Rudolf Krönlein in 1884. Krönlein published his cases in 1886. In 1884 he had diagnosed an acute abdomen as being due to either a perforated appendix or an acute intestinal obstruction. Through a midline incision he removed the appendix and did the accustomed thorough antiseptic washing out of the peritoneal cavity. The patient, a lad of seventeen, died two days later. In another case Krönlein could not find the appendix and he regarded the outlook as hopeless. However, he did his best to try and disinfect the intestines by washing them for an hour and a quarter. He then closed the abdomen without drainage and, against his expectation, the patient recovered. Krönlein acknowledged his debt to Lawson Tait who had shortly before published his account of 208 abdominal sections and had shown what the new surgery was capable of accomplishing.

A further great advance was made by T. G. Morton of Philadelphia in 1887. Morton diagnosed acute appendicitis, operated, opened an abscess, and removed the appendix with a successful result. This was the first successful appendicectomy in which the operation was primarily undertaken for the diseased appendix. Morton made the following remarks at the time:

"In the treatment of perityphlitic abscess with or without appendix perforation an incision should be made as soon as the symptoms indicate the possible or probable formation of abscess or perforation. Now that the abdominal cavity can be sectioned there should be no delay in promptly making at least an exploratory incision. The delay in such cases constitutes one of the chief sources of the well recognized great mortality."

It may be noted that in May 1886 J. R. Hall, of New York, had operated on a boy of seventeen for an inguinal hernia thought to be strangulated. The hernial sac contained a perforated appendix which was safely excised. Although the diagnosis was not made before operation, this was probably the first successful appendicectomy in a case of perforative appendicitis.

Many other American surgeons were inspired by the work of Fitz and Parker. Henry B. Sands, at one time assistant to Willard Parker, gave a valuable account of the early signs of perforation and made a strong plea for early operation. On 30 December, 1887, he saw a patient whom he recognized as suffering from peritonitis due to perforation of the appendix and he operated within forty-eight hours of the onset of acute symptoms. He found a perforated appendix with spreading peritonitis. After removing two concretions he trimmed the edges of the perforation, sutured it, washed out the wound, and drained it. The patient recovered.

Charles McBurney recounted his experience with early operative intervention in a famous paper read before the New York Surgical Society in November 1889. He described the point of maximal tenderness in acute appendicitis (McBurney's point) as follows: "I believe that in every case the seat of greatest pain determined by the pressure of one finger, has been very exactly between an inch and a half and two inches from the anterior spinous process of the ilium on a straight line drawn from that process to the umbilicus." In 1894 McBurney described his muscle-splitting or gridiron incision. He claimed that it gave a more direct approach to the appendix and reduced the risk of rupture of the incisional wound in the postoperative period.

In Great Britain progress was less rapid. Sir Frederick Treves was one of the first surgeons in this country to operate for appendicitis. In February 1887 he operated on a patient between attacks. He found a kinked appendix, divided the adhesions, and straightened it out. In the course of a subsequent discussion on this case he agreed that it would have been better to have removed the appendix and in fact he soon began the practice of appendicectomy. He became the great advocate of the "interval" operation—that is, removal of the appendix during a quiescent period—and his conservative attitude greatly influenced the practice of British surgeons. It is significant that the first book on appendicitis to be published in England did not appear until 1895 and then it was written, not by a surgeon, but by a physician, Dr. Herbert Hawkins.

The abandonment of a wait-and-see policy in the management of appendicitis and the rapid development of operative treatment were greatly influenced by the case of King Edward VII in 1902. In June of that year elaborate preparations were being made for the crowning of Edward VII when it was suddenly announced that he suffered from perityphlitis, and that the coronation was postponed. On June 13, while staying at Windsor, the royal patient had a sudden attack of abdominal pain which was diagnosed as appendicitis by Sir Francis Laking and Sir Thomas Barlow. Treves was called in consultation five days later. The temperature gradually fell and the local swelling and tenderness subsided. By June 21 the patient had sufficiently recovered to return to London. That same evening, however, there was a sudden rise of temperature and a large painful swelling appeared in the right side. The King was seen early on June 24 by Lord Lister, then in his seventy-sixth year, and by Sir Thomas Smith who advised immediate operation. Edward however was obstinate: "I must keep faith with my people and go to the Abbey." Finally, Treves said bluntly: "Then, Sir, you will go as a corpse." The operation followed at 11 a.m. Dr. Frederick Hewitt gave the anaesthetic and Treves operated upon his sovereign—a stout man and not a good surgical risk. Pus was found at a depth of four and a half inches, and two large drainage tubes were inserted, surrounded by iodoform gauze. Nothing was reported concerning the appendix itself and it was probably not disturbed. The King made an uneventful recovery. He had no further attacks of abdominal pain and died of broncho-pneumonia in 1910. No account of any post-mortem examination was issued.

Following that historic operation, appendicitis became a fashionable disease. Treves, who had borne a crushing weight of reponsibility, was created a Baronet with the augmentation of a Lion of England in his coat of arms. By a strange trick of fate Treves lost his own daughter from perforative appendicitis —no operation being attempted—and he himself died of peritonitis in 1923.

A few other landmarks in the history of the surgery of acute abdominal emergencies may be mentioned. In 1883 Lawson Tait, whose prowess as an ovariotomist has already been noticed, performed the first successful operation for a ruptured extra-uterine gestation. Ectopic or extra-uterine pregnancy occurs when the fertilized ovum fails to reach the uterus, but becomes embedded and develops in some part of the Fallopian tube*—the tube which connects the ovary with the uterus. Very rarely, extra-uterine pregnancy occurs in the ovary and still more rarely in the peritoneum. When pregnancy occurs in the Fallopian tube the ovum usually separates from the maternal structures and this separation is accompanied by haemorrhage. The haemorrhage in turn causes a rupture of the tube and blood flows into the peritoneal cavity; in some

* So named after Gabriel Fallopius (1523–62), Professor of Anatomy at Padua, who gave the earliest accurate description of these tubes or oviducts.

cases the blood rapidly fills up the pelvis. Before 1883 nearly all the victims of this disaster bled to death, because no one thought it was possible to deal with such a crisis at the time of the rupture. It had been suggested that the only way in which a woman dying from rupture of an extra-uterine pregnancy could be saved would be to open the abdomen, tie the bleeding vessels, and remove the products of conception; but no one before Lawson Tait had attempted to do this. Tait had seen more than a score of these tragic cases, but in spite of the extraordinary success of his other abdominal operations he was very reluctant to intervene with the knife. Finally, in January 1883, he did operate; but the patient was seen too late and she did not survive. Two months later Tait was called in consultation to another case of the same kind, on this occasion he did not hesitate. "I advised abdominal section and found the abdomen full of clot. The right Fallopian tube was ruptured and from it a placenta was protruding. I tied the tube and removed it. I searched for, but could not find the foetus, and I suppose it got lost amongst the folds of the intestines and there was absorbed. Certainly it has not been seen since. The patient made a very protracted convalescence but she is now perfectly well."

One of the commonest of abdominal emergencies is rupture of a gastric or duodenal ulcer. As with a ruptured extra-uterine pregnancy, early operation offers the only hope for the patient. Until almost the end of the nineteenth century this hope was denied the many victims of this catastrophe. In 1884 the German surgeon von Mikulicz faced up to the issue and argued that "every physician and surgeon must consider the question whether in cases of stomach or intestinal perforation one ought to open the abdomen, suture the perforation, and by a thorough cleansing of the peritoneal cavity try to stop the threatening or already begun peritonitis". Several unsuccessful attempts to save patients suffering from a perforated ulcer were made from 1885 onwards, but the first victory over this agonizingly painful and invariably fatal condition was not won until 19 May, 1892. On that day a man of forty-one who had suffered from indigestion for many years and had had several haemorrhages was awakened at two o'clock in the morning by a sudden attack of acute pain in the region of the stomach. The patient's doctor was called at four o'clock and Ludwig Heusner, a surgeon of Barmen, was summoned later in the day. Heusner was away from home and had to be recalled by telegram, but he eventually arrived and confirmed the diagnosis of an acute perforation. The patient could not be moved; there were no proper facilities for carrying out the antiseptic technique and the lighting was abominable. Nevertheless, Heusner knew that immediate intervention offered the only chance of saving the patient's life and at 6.30 p.m. he began the operation. It lasted two and a half hours! A perforation of the stomach was found after a long search and sutured with great difficulty. Blood and stomach contents were mopped out with gauze and the abdominal wall was closed with thick silk sutures. The patient made an uninterrupted recovery.

The first successful British case of the same kind was that of Mr. Hastings Gilford of Reading on 22 June, 1893, and the second that of Thomas Morse of Norwich who, on 7 December, 1893, operated upon a twenty-year-old girl five and a half hours after perforation. Morse's operation was, like that of Heusner, performed in a private house, and a notable feature of it was that after the hole in the stomach had been closed the abdomen was washed out with seventeen pints of hot water. By 1896 the operation for suture of a perforated gastric or duodenal ulcer had been established as a standard procedure.

The surgery of the brain, the spinal cord and the chest developed later than that of the abdomen. Although trephination of the skull had been practised since the Stone Age (see page 20), no advances in the surgery of the brain itself were made until the last quarter of the nineteenth century. Before that time little was known about the functions of the various parts of the brain; there was even uncertainty as to which parts were essential to life. The work of Sir David Ferrier, Sir Charles Sherrington, and the great Russian physiologist Pavlov, laid the foundations of all modern conceptions of cerebral function and paved the way for the neurosurgeon.

On 25 November, 1884, a tumour of the brain was first successfully diagnosed during life, accurately localized, and removed by operation. The patient, a man of twenty-five, was diagnosed by Dr. Alexander Hughes Bennett as having a tumour of the brain and he was admitted into the Hospital for Epilepsy and Paralysis in Regent's Park. The tumour was thought to be located in the cortex near to a structure known as the fissure of Rolando.* The patient was very anxious to have it removed, and Mr. (later Sir) Rickman Godlee,† one of the consultants to the hospital, was called upon to operate. The skull was opened and the brain exposed. The preoperative localization proved to be accurate and a tumour the size of a walnut was removed without difficulty. The case aroused great public interest and, as the patient lived for only a month, an outcry was raised in some quarters that the operation was unjustified. It was however, generally agreed that a great advance had been made in regard to surgical interference with the human brain, and within a few years successful operations in cases of cerebral tumours were being carried out in many countries.

The real founder of neurosurgery in England was Sir Victor Horsley, surgeon to University College Hospital and to the National Hospital for Nervous Diseases in Queen Square. Horsley was an experimental physiologist as well as a surgeon and he made valuable contributions to the knowledge of localization of cerebral function. But even when a considerable amount of knowledge had been acquired regarding the structure and functions of the brain, many technical difficulties had to be surmounted before operations on that organ could be undertaken with any degree of safety. One of the main difficulties was the control of haemorrhage from the cranial bones, which was often severe. Horsley solved this problem when he discovered that bleeding from the raw edges of the cut bones could be controlled by smearing them with modelling wax that had been rendered antiseptic. At a much later

---

* So named after Luigi Rolando (1773–1831), Professor of Anatomy at Turin, who first described this fissure between the parietal and frontal lobes of the brain.

† Sir Rickman John Godlee (1849–1925) was a nephew of Lord Lister. He became Surgeon-in-Ordinary to Edward VII and George V and President of the Royal College of Surgeons.

date (1914) Horsley found that troublesome haemorrhage from the brain itself could often be controlled by the close application of living muscle tissue to the bleeding surface.

The pioneers of brain surgery used the simple trephine for the purpose of opening the cranium, but later electrically driven perforators and burrs were also employed. Considerable use was also made of Gigli's wire saw for cutting the bridges of bone left between the holes bored by the trephine. This ingenious instrument consisted of a piano-wire with a screw-thread turned on it and with handles which could be attached at each end. The saw was passed by means of a probe under the bone from one opening to another.

On 9 June, 1887, Mr. Victor Horsley (as he then was) performed the first successful operation for removal of a tumour of the spinal cord. The patient was an army officer of forty-two who had for three years been affected with partial paralysis of the bladder and complete paralysis of the legs. He suffered frightful pain and unless given some relief he could not long survive. Dr. (later Sir) William Gowers, the leading neurologist of the day, had examined the patient and had ascribed the symptoms to a tumour high up in the spinal cord. Horsley operated and succeeded in removing the tumour. Twelve months later the patient was in excellent health and he remained well up to the time of his death from another cause some twenty years after the operation.

Sir William Macewen, Professor of Surgery at Glasgow, was also a great pioneer of brain surgery. In 1893 he published a classical work entitled *Pyogenic Infective Diseases of the Brain and Spinal Cord*. In this book he gave extensive reports on sixty-five patients upon whom he had operated for brain abscesses. As early as 1879 he had successfully removed a tumour of the dura mater, the membranous envelope which covers the brain and spinal cord, and he had also operated for the treatment of intracranial haemorrhage.

During the last quarter of the century surgeons began for the first time to perform extensive operations within the thorax. In this field also Sir William Macewen was an outstanding leader. In 1895 Sir William Tennant Gairdner, one of his colleagues at the Glasgow Western Infirmary, asked Macewen to take over from his medical ward a very serious case of unilateral tuberculosis of the lung. Gairdner was convinced that only surgery could help the patient, but he did not think that anything more than a purely palliative operation was possible. Macewen removed the whole of the left lung, and the patient lived to a ripe old age after a life of normal activity. Some little time after the discharge of his patient Macewen was walking home one night when he thought he recognized the voice of a man who was discoursing loudly to a little group of people standing in the light of a fog-enshrouded street lamp. On going closer he saw that it was a Salvation Army meeting and that it was his former patient who was holding forth. Macewen waited until the meeting finished and then told the Salvationist that open-air preaching was an activity in which a man with one lung could not safely indulge.

Artificial pneumothorax for the treatment of consumption was first induced by the Italian physician Carlo Forlanini in 1888. This procedure, which was designed to collapse and give rest to the affected lung, had been suggested by James Carson, a Liverpool surgeon, in 1822. Thoracotomy (incision into the thorax) for the evacuation of pus was first carried out by Ernst Küstner in 1889. The first thoracoplasty was done by George Ryerson Fowler of New York in 1893 and decortication (stripping the thickened pleura from the lung) for the treatment of chronic empyema was introduced by Edmond Delorme in 1894. The first successful suture of the heart was done by L. Rehn of Frankfort in 1896.

On 15 March, 1849, Dr. Thomas Addison of Guy's Hospital read before the South London Medical Society a paper in which he described the condition which is now known as "Addison's disease". He showed that the condition was caused by disease of the suprarenal glands and provided the first evidence that these minute bodies situated near the upper end of each kidney were essential to life. Addison's observations inaugurated the modern study of the endocrine or ductless glands and of their secretions—the mysterious hormones or chemical messengers which regulate many of the most important functions of the body. It has indeed been said that the whole of the vast modern science of endocrinology dates from

15 March, 1849. Surgery of the endocrine glands is—with the exception of the thyroid—a comparatively recent development. The thyroid had long been a subject of investigation and years before anything was known about hormones several physicians had noted the coincidence of various disease conditions with enlargement of the gland.

The thyroid was the first of the endocrine glands to receive attention from the surgeon; it is indeed probable that goitre was treated surgically in the time of the ancient Greeks. In more modern times Mr. Joseph Henry Green, of St. Thomas's Hospital, is credited with the removal of the right lobe of the thyroid as early as 1828, his patient dying fifteen days later from sepsis. The first total excision of the gland was probably carried out by Paul Sick, a German surgeon, in 1867. In 1874 Sir Patrick Heron Watson, senior surgeon to the Edinburgh Royal Infirmary, reported a case of excision of the thyroid in the treatment of goitre. The greatest pioneer of thyroidectomy was, however, Theodor Kocher, a pupil of Billroth, who was for many years Professor of Surgery at Berne in Switzerland. Kocher performed his first thyroidectomy for goitre in 1878; by the time of his death in 1917 he had performed this difficult operation over 2,000 times with a mortality rate of only 4½ per cent.

In the present century the surgery of the endocrine glands has assumed tremendous importance. Many serious diseases caused by dysfunction of the pituitary, the parathyroids, the suprarenals, the pancreas, the pineal gland, and the thymus have yielded to direct surgical attack upon the glands themselves.

The surgical treatment of enlargement of the prostate gland was inaugurated by the Italian Enrico Bottini and the American surgeon Eugene Fuller in the 1890s. The man who did most to popularize the operation was Sir Peter Freyer, of the Indian Medical Service. The treatment of diseases of bones and joints was greatly advanced by Hugh Owen Thomas (1834–91) of Liverpool and by his nephew and pupil, Sir Robert Jones.

Writing in 1874 Sir John Eric Erichsen, Professor of Surgery at University College, London, predicted that "the abdomen, the chest, and the brain would be for ever shut from the intrusions of the wise and humane surgeon". Within twenty years of this pronouncement surgeons had successfully removed the stomach and large parts of the intestines, a whole lung had been excised, and a brain tumour had been extirpated. These operations were not mere feats of surgical showmanship; they saved the lives and restored the health of thousands of human beings. Although it is true that these great accomplishments, and all the triumphs of present-day surgery, were made possible by the introduction of anaesthesia and antisepsis a mere century ago, every surgeon and every patient owes an incalculable debt to those masters of the more distant past who laid the foundations of the art and science of surgery.

FOR FURTHER READING

Bailey, H. and Bishop, W. J. *Notable Names in Medicine and Surgery.* 3rd ed. 1959.

Bett, W. R. *The History and Conquest of Common Diseases.* Norman, Oklahoma. 1954.

Bowman, A. K. *The Life and Teaching of Sir William Macewen.* 1942.

Cope, Sir Z. *Pioneers in Acute Abdominal Surgery.* 1939.

Crowe, S. T. *Halsted of Johns Hopkins, the Man and his Men.* Springfield, Ill. 1957.

Flack, I. H. *Lawson Tait, 1845–1899.* 1949.

Garrison, F. H. *An Introduction to the History of Medicine.* 4th ed. Philadelphia. 1929.

Le Vay, D. *The Life of Hugh Owen Thomas.* Edinburgh. 1956.

MacKay, W. J. *Lawson Tait, his Life and Work.* 1922.

Paget, S. *Sir Victor Horsley: A Study of his Life and Work.* 1919.

Rolleston, Sir H. *The Endocrine Organs in Health and Disease.* 1936.

Watson, F. *The Life of Sir Robert Jones.* 1934.

Index

Abbott, Gilbert, 160
Abdomen, wounds and injuries of, 16, 19, 39, 51, 67, 73
Abdominal surgery, 43, 144, 149, 150, 172, 174, 175, 180, 181
Abernethy, John, 122, 135, 142
Acupuncture, 41
Addison, Thomas, 144, 184
Aesculapius, 47
Aetius of Amida, 56
Agatha, Saint, 58
Albucasis, 72, 73, 83
Alexander of Tralles, 56
Alexandria, medical school of, 50
Ambulances, 70, 145
American Civil War, 131, 152
American Indians, 14, 26
Amputation, 43, 44, 52, 54, 70, 73, 82, 92, 95–7, 105, 117, 122, 133, 136, 137, 143, 144, 145, 146, 147
  by primitives, 26, 28
  flap method, 52, 96, 97
Amyand, Claudius, 124, 125, 126
Anaesthesia, 40, 42, 43, 59, 60, 62, 131, 143, 155–62
  local, 173
  refrigeration, 146
Anal fistula, 38, 43, 67, 111
Anatomy, 66, 72, 76, 77, 78, 86, 112
  teaching of, 50, 65, 76, 86, 89, 90, 110, 111, 141
Anatomy Act, 140
Anderson, Thomas, 166
Anel, Dominique, 116
Aneurysm, 54, 73, 116, 135, 142
Anthrax, 165
Antiseptic system, 62, 165–9, 174
Ants, suturing by means of, 15, 39, 67, 73
Antyllus, 54
Aorta, abdominal, ligation of, 135, 136
Apollonia, Saint, 58
Apothecaries, 90
Appendicitis, 123, 124, 126, 144, 175–179
Apprenticeship, 88, 89, 120
Arabic surgery, 71–4
Archigenes, 52
Arderne, John of, 67, 68
Aretaeus, 123
Arnold of Villanova, 60

Arrow wounds, 15, 16, 43, 46, 47, 62, 70
Artery clamps, 174
Arthritis, 11, 12
Asepsis, 168, 169
Assyrian surgery, 30, 35, 36
Astrology, 61
Atherstone, W. G., 161
Australian aborigines, 12, 14, 15, 18
Aveling, J. H., 153
Avicenna, 72

Babylonian surgery, 30, 35, 36
Bacteria, 11, 163–5
Bandaging, 18, 33, 37, 117, 145
Banester, John, 90
Barber-surgeons, 36, 65, 86, 87, 88, 89, 90, 93
Barber-Surgeons' Company, 87, 88, 89, 90, 93, 110, 111, 120
Barlow, Sir Thomas, 178
Bell, Benjamin, 123
Bell, Sir Charles, 140, 141, 142
Bell, John, 140, 141, 150
Belloste, Augustin, 117
Bennett, Alexander Hughes, 182
Bergmann, Ernst von, 168, 169
Bernard de Gordon, 60
Bible, surgery in the, 44
Bigelow, Henry Jacob, 161, 170
Bigelow, Jacob, 161
Billroth, Theodor, 172
Blaise, Saint, 58
Blood-letting, 18, 28, 44, 61, 63, 148
Blood transfusion, 108, 112–15, 151–3, 156
Blood vessels, ligation of, 14, 38, 41, 51
Blundell, James, 151, 152
Body-snatching, 123
Bone, diseases of, 11, 12, 18, 185
Boott, Francis, 161
Bottini, Enrico, 185
Boyer, Alexis, 148, 149
Bradwell, Stephen, 98
Braid, James, 157, 158
Brain surgery, 181–3
Brancas, 85
Breast, amputation of, 56
  cancer of, 51, 173
  plastic surgery of, 83

187

188 INDEX

Surgery, after Lister—*cont.*
Japanese, 43
medieval, 58–75
of Ancient East, 30–45
prehistoric, 12, 13
primitive, 13–29
Renaissance, 76–94
Roman, 55–7
Tudor, 86–94
Susruta, 37, 38, 39, 40
Sutton, Daniel, 126
Sutures and suturing, 14, 15, 38, 53, 67, 72, 73, 146
Syme, James, 135, 144, 167
Symonds, Sir Charters, 175
Sympathetic magic, 81, 103, 104

Tagliacozzi, Gaspare, 85, 86
Tait, Robert Lawson, 175, 176, 179, 180
Talmud, 44
Tamba, Yasuhori, 43
Taylor, Chevalier, 128
Temple healing, 47, 48
Tendons, suture of, 106
Tetanus, 68
Theodoric of Cervia, 62
Thermometer, clinical, 131
Thiersch, Karl, 172
Thomas, Hugh Owen, 185
Thoracic surgery, 183, 184
Thoracoplasty, 184
Thoracotomy, 184
Thorns, suturing by means of, 15
Thymus gland, 137
Thyroid gland, 185
Tibet, 26
Tilanus, C. B., 148, 149
Tonsillectomy, 38, 51, 56, 129, 130
Tourniquet, 116, 172
Tracheotomy, 85
Travers, Benjamin, 135, 143

Trephination, 44, 49, 51, 56, 63, 73, 107, 129, 181
in Ancient Egypt, 33
prehistoric, 20–2
primitive, 22–4
Treves, Sir Frederick, 179, 180
Trusses, 66, 127
Tuberculosis, 12, 98, 121

Vaccination, 126
Van Bortel, 128
Varicose veins, 48, 49, 50
Venesection, 18
Vesalius, Andreas, 77, 78
Vesico-vaginal fistula, 170
Vicary, Thomas, 86, 87
Vigo, John of, 79, 84, 85
Vivisection, human, 50, 65, 66
Volkmann, Richard von, 168, 172
Votive offerings, 48

Wallis, Robert, 88
Warren, John Collins, 160
Watson, Sir Patrick Heron, 185
Watson, Sir Thomas, 173
Weapon salve, 103, 104
Weise, Martin, 108
Wells, Horace, 160
Wells, Sir Thomas Spencer, 174, 175
White, Charles, 122
Wiseman, Richard, 98, 99, 100, 101, 102, 103
Woelfler, Anton, 172
Woodall, John, 92, 95
Wound treatment, 28, 78, 79, 116
primitive, 13–19
Wren, Sir Christopher, 108, 113

Yin Chung k'an, 41
Yonge, James, 96, 97
Yu Fu, 41